CW01370106

Milton Keynes UK
Ingram Content Group UK Ltd.
UKHW032331231124
451543UK00013B/446

"Based on Will Parfitt's forty years of practice as a psychosynthesis psychotherapist and trainer and the distance course he created, this book is indeed a precious gift. Its content is unique; reading it, one truly has the impression of being accompanied with wisdom by Parfitt's friendly voice on the journey of Psychosynthesis and the fuller journey of Life."

Petra Guggisberg Nocelli, Trainer at the Institute of Psychosynthesis in Italy, and author of several books including *The Way of Psychosynthesis* and the 2-volume *Know, Love, Transform Yourself.*

"In this splendid book Will presents a comprehensive, insightful, and holistic overview of Psychosynthesis as a model for self-knowledge, providing a blueprint for Self-realisation. Not for the faint of heart, the reader is invited on a journey that promises transformative experiences and outcomes that will enrich the depth of fulfilment and meaning of their lives."

Diana Whitmore, Founder and CoCEO of Growing2gether, founder of the Psychosynthesis Trust and author of *Psychosynthesis in Education: the Joy of Learning* and *Psychosynthesis Counselling in Action.*

"An in-depth and practical guide that seamlessly combines theory and practice within psychosynthesis, Parfitt's wisdom and personal account of his path to psychosynthesis adds an authentic and engaging tone to the book. He excels at presenting complex ideas in an understandable way, making the book accessible to both beginners and more experienced practitioners of psychosynthesis. Parfitt's insightful approach makes this book a unique, inspiring and invaluable guide on the path toward self-realization and inner harmony."

Mats Graffman, Executive Director of Humanova, a leading authority in the Nordics for personal development and leadership training based on psychosynthesis.

"Another gem from Will Parfitt, written with his customary luminous clarity and readable style. His vocation as a teacher shines through the text as he accompanies the reader on a journey of discovery—through

terrain intimate and personal, and also realms transpersonal and philosophical. Practical exercises, thoughtful insights and warm encouragement are offered throughout."
> **Melanie Reinhart**, Author of *Chiron and the Healing Journey*, internationally renowned astrologer and Patron of the Faculty of Astrological Studies [UK]

"Will Parfitt has more than four decades of experience in the wide field of psychology, psychosynthesis, Kabbalah and esoteric wisdom and is an excellent teacher and author. In this book he shows a profound way for people interested in self-empowerment or who long for a soulful, visionary and fulfilled life. I highly recommend this book to everybody who is willing to follow their path on their soul journey."
> **Gerhard Singer-Schobel**, Founder and head of The Swiss psychosynthesis training aeon, certified trainer, supervisor and teaching therapist in psychosynthesis and other modalities.

"Written in a very clear and inviting style which is born out of the writer's in-depth personal and professional journey, this is a wonderful guide to self-development. Taking one delightful step at a time, the reader is invited on a journey of discovery which is profoundly articulate, yet simple and easy to follow. This is a book which I will return to in different times of need. It has a structure and subtle mastery which can only be achieved through the writer having lived and breathed the essence of psychosynthesis. A wonderful, full and rich adventure awaits the reader."
> **Kim Shiller**, Programme Director, Psychosynthesis Trust, London

"The author has impressively succeeded in clearly demonstrating the essence of psychosynthesis and translating it into contemporary language. Numerous exercises, followed by valuable explanations to help us understand our own symbols and experiences, assist on this journey of discovery and connects us ever more deeply with the essence of ourselves which seeks expression in the world. This book is a valuable companion for our journey to the true self."
> **Mirjam Lauber**, Founder of the Psychosynthesis Training in Brig-Glis, and Zürich, Switzerland, organisational coach and teacher of process-oriented centering.

"This book will guide you on a journey to the centre of your true self. As a traveller on this path you will be encouraged at each stage of the journey to gently open, like a flower, to your unique wholeness. It's a journey to be savoured, not rushed, with breaks built into the route allowing time to review and consolidate what is encountered along the way."

Joyce Hopewell, Former Principal of the English Huber School, author of several books including *Piercing the Egg Shell* and *The Second Time Around*.

"Will's use of straightforward and understandable language makes psychosynthesis accessible to those with no background in the subject, as well as for us "old-timers" who (like myself) may be surprised at new ways of seeing. I heartily recommend this book for anyone looking to deepen their understanding of psychosynthesis or simply taking the journey for the first time."

Marjorie Hope Gross, Holistic Counsellor and Coach, past co-chair of the Association for the Advancement of Psychosynthesis and editor of Psychosynthesis Quarterly.

THE JOURNEY
OF PSYCHOSYNTHESIS

Also by Will Parfitt

PSYCHOLOGY

The Magic of Psychosynthesis: Initiation and Self-Development
The Something and Nothing of Death

KABBALAH

Kabbalah: The Tree of Life [illustrated]
Kabbalah For Life
The Complete Guide to the Kabbalah

FICTION

Rose of Heaven
Meetings With Amazing People
This Beautiful Garden

THE JOURNEY OF PSYCHOSYNTHESIS

Lessons in Self-Awareness and Making Your Best Choices

Will Parfitt

AEON

First published in 2024 by
Aeon Books

Copyright © 2024 by Will Parfitt

The right of Will Parfitt to be identified as the author of this work has been asserted in accordance with §§ 77 and 78 of the Copyright Design and Patents Act 1988.

All rights reserved. No part of this publication may be reproduced, stored in a retrieval system, or transmitted, in any form or by any means, electronic, mechanical, photocopying, recording, or otherwise, without the prior written permission of the publisher.

British Library Cataloguing in Publication Data

A C.I.P. for this book is available from the British Library

ISBN-13: 978-1-80152-143-7

Cover photograph by Will Parfitt
Typeset by Medlar Publishing Solutions Pvt Ltd, India

www.aeonbooks.co.uk

CONTENTS

Acknowledgements   vii

Introduction   1

How to effectively use the lessons   5

LESSON 1
The journey of life: a process of cycles within cycles   11

LESSON 2
Models of awareness: understanding our inner world   27

LESSON 3
Subpersonalities and self-expression: exploring our many roles   47

LESSON 4
Love and relationship: towards balance and harmony within   63

LESSON 5
The child of wisdom: the inner child and family dynamics   81

LESSON 6
The art of self-identification: becoming the conductor
    of your life   99

LESSON 7
The power of imagination: living within the world we create   119

LESSON 8
Purpose and the process of willing: personal and spiritual
    empowerment   137

LESSON 9
The realms of spirit and shadow: exploring the heights
    and depths of the psyche   157

LESSON 10
Acceptance and change: global issues and embodying
    leadership   179

AFTERWORD
The wisdom of psychosynthesis   201

APPENDIX 1
Further reading and training   203

APPENDIX 2
A book map   209

Index   215

ACKNOWLEDGEMENTS

Firstly, to all the students and graduates of the distance courses that made the lessons themselves, and subsequently this book, enjoyable to create and effective in practice.

Secondly, to all the people who have supported my own journey of psychosynthesis, especially those who in one way or another supported the creation and continuation of the distance learning programme, most notably: Patti Howe, Diana Whitmore, Joan Wenske, Pat Jones, Tim Owen, Debra Galpin, Meir Spungin, Ewa Robertson, Chris Robertson, Jane Mayers, Mirjam Lauber, and Barbara Landis.

Disclaimer
The information herein is not a substitute for professional medical or legal care or advice. The author does not assume responsibility for your thoughts, decisions, or actions.

Introduction

Back in the mid-1970s I had no idea how my future would unfold. After several years involved in esoteric and occult research and practice, I felt somewhat disillusioned—not so much by the more abstract or inner-orientated practices and beliefs I held, but more by the unconscious acting out of unresolved psychological issues by myself and my peers. The only group that I belonged to that made any sense to me insisted on no personal interactions, but that wasn't enough to assuage my thirst for meaningful daily relating beyond idle chatter.

Then I discovered the human potential movement and my life was transformed. By around 1978 I was very involved and attending many different gestalt, rebirthing and bioenergetic growth groups. Life seemed so much more open and engaging, but I still had a sense of something missing. A wise mentor who knew of my previous history with esoteric and spiritual practices told me how psychosynthesis married the best psychological methods with transpersonal practices and pointed me in that direction.

The very next weekend I attended my first introduction to psychosynthesis with Diana Whitmore (or Becchetti as she still was then). It was a wonderful course and it set me on a track to the future. I realised that I had found the path I had been searching for, one that integrated the psychological with the spiritual in a way that segued perfectly with my esoteric knowledge and practice. I set out on my journey of psychosynthesis and had the good fortune to be with a fantastic trainer who chose me to be one of her apprentices, an elevated role that had its shadow as well as bright side, but offered me the wonderful opportunity to learn, to practise and to teach psychosynthesis.

An Italian doctor, Roberto Assagioli, founded psychosynthesis in the mid-20th century. He had trained as a psychoanalyst but also had a deep interest in esoteric and mystical practices. The more he worked with people in the analytical mode, the more he felt there was something missing, some vital aspects of the person that were not being honoured or addressed—the transpersonal realms of spiritual understanding, wisdom, love, and inspiration. You can see why I was immediately taken with this approach. Assagioli once said that psychoanalysis was primarily concerned with the basement of the psyche whereas psychosynthesis is concerned with the whole building. Once we learn to access the whole building, it is then possible to include all aspects of ourselves and we can live in a more holistic way.

Modern counsellors and psychotherapists, whatever their discipline, take the role that was once ascribed to the "wise person" or "shaman". They are expected to have an understanding of the inner world and to be able to use this understanding to heal people. Psychosynthesis, by including the spirit and soul, allows a thorough holistic healing to take place. It also has a connection to esoteric traditions that are much older than modern psychology and gives practitioners something to lean into in support of their work.

Psychosynthesis does not only teach you how to work with other people, though. Many who train in psychosynthesis do that, but the majority of people who undertake psychosynthesis either as a training, with an individual guide, or through a course such as in this book, then utilise psychosynthesis for their personal development or in their own field of work. This includes education, medicine, social work, the arts, engineering—you name it and the principles of psychosynthesis can be applied to it.

All the signs suggest that psychosynthesis is continuing to grow, for unlike some other similar methods for personal understanding, it is not a finished system but one that is willing to change and grow as the world changes and grows. Nurturing a deeper connection with our spiritual core intensifies our ability to shed light in our surroundings, transform our environment, and live with a new depth of understanding and creativity. We create the world in which we live through our imagination and our will, properly tempered by love, the force by which we maintain it.

Back in those, for me, heady days of the late 1970s, however, I didn't know where this training would lead me and would have been disbelieving if I had been told I would be spending the following forty or so years working as a psychosynthesis therapist and supervisor, teaching psychosynthesis internationally, running a distance learning programme with hundreds of students and writing several books on the subject.

During my early years in psychosynthesis, I was aware of how there were people who for various reasons couldn't attend training courses, and might find it difficult to find an individual practitioner. In 1990, *The Elements of Psychosynthesis*, my first book on the subject, came out and sold extremely well, proving to me the interest was certainly there. I realised the solution could be a distance learning course, and here you are, more than thirty years later, with an updated version of the course in your hands.

The content of this book, then, is unique, being based on a long-term tried and tested course in psychosynthesis that has spanned more than two decades. The course had a wide range of students hailing from various corners of the world, encompassing diverse backgrounds and beliefs, and over half of whom were female. A majority of students reported that the course had a powerful impact and an enduring relevance in their lives.

The aim is to make psychosynthesis relatable to your everyday life and to present the content in easy-to-understand language. The lessons offer you ways to discover more about yourself and increase your self-awareness to enable a more fulfilling life, and to connect you to the power of the will and improve your life choices. As you will learn, though, psychosynthesis is not about the application of techniques, but learning to live with a vision that comes from deep within oneself.

How to effectively use the lessons

You could do the lessons in this book without reading these instructions, and some people will undoubtedly do so. However, you'll find it much easier if you spend a while reading the suggestions—nothing is too complicated and, once you start the work, you'll find the lessons flow easily. Also, of course, once you are in the swing of the work, you'll develop your own approach and level of engagement—which is as it should be. Nothing here is set in stone; once you have the basics of psychosynthesis, you primarily work with what emerges from inside you, not through following some preset plan.

Approaching the lessons

- Before starting a lesson, glance through the whole chapter to get an overall feel of it;
- follow the material in the order given;
- if you want to repeat exercises more than once, please do;
- be aware of any sensations, feelings, thoughts, insights, and resistances that emerge, particularly when doing exercises;

- record all relevant material in your journal (more on this later);
- after you finish a chapter, run back through it to check what you have taken in, what missed, what you need to spend more time with, and so on.

Preparation for exercises and other activities

You will find the words "after preparation" at the beginning of some of the activities and exercises described in the lessons. Gauge how much to do depending upon your own nature and what is being specifically asked of you in the particular exercise. Don't skimp on the time taken to do preparation work—it is a vital part of your development.

Of foremost importance in your preparation is to "relax and centre". You can do this any way you choose, and throughout this course you will learn new techniques for both relaxing and centring yourself. The more relaxed you are, the easier it will be to do the exercises, and the more you will get from them. You need to be able to relax both your mind and body to be in a fully relaxed state.

Relaxing the body can be achieved in many ways. Well-known and effective is the technique whereby you relax each part of the body in turn, beginning with your toes and moving slowly up to the top of your head (or vice versa). By focusing awareness on a part of the body, feeling its tenseness, then consciously choosing to relax, you can work over the whole body and end up feeling very relaxed. Do not fall asleep, however!

Relaxing your mind is not always so easy. A fairly effective method is to imagine your mind full of the waves of a choppy sea, which slowly becomes calmer and calmer until it is a still pool of water, untouched by any disturbances. Any thoughts that then arise can be allowed to send a ripple over the water but without disturbing its overriding serenity. You can devise other similar images to accomplish the same effect.

A good technique for overall relaxation is to suggest to yourself that you will relax in body and mind when you focus your attention on a symbol. You can choose any symbol for this; for example, a candle flame, a butterfly, a particular place you associate with relaxation, a falling leaf. Focus your attention on your breathing, then visualise your chosen symbol, knowing that focusing on it will bring relaxation. This auto-suggestive method of relaxation can be highly effective.

Simply paying attention to your breathing, watching the tide of breath entering and leaving your body, is another simple way to relax.

Some people aid their relaxation by focusing on their breathing in this way, then counting backwards from ten to one, affirming that they will be completely relaxed when they reach the number one. This also works, but remember, if you do this, to count yourself back up to ten when you finish your work.

Taking breaks

Throughout the lessons, you will come across "¶ BREAK", which represents the end of a section. When you meet this symbol, it is time to take a break. This break may be short, or may signify a break between study periods; this will depend upon your unique way of working. Don't rush the work, give it time to sink in; at the same time, don't go so slow you lose touch with the momentum of the work. As an indicator, I think a lesson should take some weeks to complete. If you did it all in a few days you may well be going too fast; in three months and you might be going too slow. Again, it does depend upon your own pace and your life circumstances.

Exercises

To help you maximise the beneficial effects of any exercise in this book, always try to make sure you have enough time to complete it without being disturbed. Even if you can only spend a very short time on a particular exercise, do set aside a specific period for it and stick to that.

Always take your time with an exercise—it is better to err on the side of slowness rather than rushing through it.

At times during exercises, you will see an ellipsis, that is, a row of three closed-up dots (...). This indicates it is a moment to take time to follow the instructions or to stay with the energies being stirred up by the work. How long for you to pause is up to you, but don't rush, take your time and the exercises will benefit you most.

It may be necessary, particularly with a longer exercise, to read it through a few times to familiarise yourself with what you have to do. Do not begrudge this time: it will help you connect with the "essence" of the exercise, and help you become focused. Some of the exercises could be recorded, thus enabling repeated use of them without interruption. This is particularly useful for long visualisations. Alternatively, of course, you could work with someone else, alternating between roles of "guide" and "explorer".

If you find any exercise particularly useful for you, stick to it for some time, even if you do not notice immediate results. Repetition of an exercise multiplies its power. Alternatively, if you find a particular exercise genuinely difficult, it may be better to leave it and return to it at another time. Do not worry if you find some of the concepts or exercises particularly difficult to understand. If this occurs you have to decide what is best for you, whether to pass on to the next part of the lesson, perhaps deciding to return later to the difficult activity, or whether for you it would be best to stick with it, using your personal power to work through this part. Whatever you decide, remember that learning can be fun despite much of what you probably experienced in school. Don't treat yourself or the work too seriously. Humour is one of our greatest teachers.

A note on visualisation

Some people find "visualisation" difficult, saying that they see no images or do not get a clear picture. That is fine! Visualisation is an unfortunate word because it suggests something "visual". In fact, for these types of exercises, many people actually "see" very little. What is more important is to get a sense of whatever it is you are being asked to do. Allow your other senses to be present: feel it, sense it. You can very effectively imagine yourself on, say, a mountain top without actually "seeing" anything.

Keeping a journal

Before actually commencing the work of the first lesson you need to acquire a suitable journal. You can use a computer word-processor to create your journal; a notebook app can be enough, or you can purchase many different journal/diary apps. Alternatively, a loose-leaf folder ring binder is an ideal "physical journal", which allows you to add or remove pages; or you could keep a digital audio journal.

It is not essential that during this course you keep a psychosynthesis journal, but it is of great benefit to do so. If you're like me, you'll feel an instant resistance to this. If you really don't want to do it, that's fine, but if you do, you will find it helps ground the learning from the activity and support your ongoing development.

You can use your journal to record:

- your practical work, including a description of any conditions you feel are significant;
- a description of relevant experiences you may have, positive or negative in nature;
- thoughts, flashes, creative insights;
- anything else you wish to include.

Keeping a journal will help you to formulate more precisely what you know (and the questions you need to ask); help make your knowledge more accessible and increase your understanding; help you make choices; call into play a sense of values, and keep your work in perspective; attune your intuition and abstract mental processes; be an act of affirmation and commitment, thus strengthening your purpose; help you see long-term trends in your growth; aid your memory; and record both successes and difficulties.

For some exercises you could introduce drawing and colour. This is not obligatory but if you choose to do so, you will need to purchase (if you don't have them already) a set of coloured pencils and pens, and any other art materials you wish. This is where a loose-leaf binder can be very useful. Alternatively, if you have such skills, you can do your artwork on a computer. If you do choose to do any artwork, remember it is not about producing great art but is a way of furthering your inner exploration.

You can write in your journal whenever you wish, but at specific times during the lessons (usually at the end of exercises, but not always) you will find the instruction [write]—this indicates that this is a good time to make an entry in your journal. Where possible, it is usually a good idea to record your experiences immediately after finishing with an exercise.

Remember, do not gossip about your work with your family or friends, or prematurely share insights, as this can dissipate the energy. But do talk about it when appropriate if it supports you in your development, or you feel a real need to do so.

LESSON 1

The journey of life: a process of cycles within cycles

In the quest for self-realisation and meaningful existence, the transformative potential of psychosynthesis can illuminate the path. Our unique creative potential is brought to life, as is our ability to function harmoniously in the world and improve the quality of all our relationships.

What makes psychosynthesis unique is that it is a distinctive fusion of principles and practices from transpersonal therapies, humanistic psychology, and spiritual traditions, resulting in a heart-centred, integrative, and holistic psychology that addresses our spiritual, emotional, mental, and physical needs. It is an open, non-dogmatic approach to personal and spiritual development that encourages you to traverse your unique path while staying true to your ethical and spiritual values.

Each of us perceives and interacts with the world through a unique lens shaped by our past and early experiences. Psychosynthesis asserts that within each individual there also resides a potential—a "future"—awaiting discovery. It restores a balance between the various parts of the personality and helps us to establish a deep connection to our core Self. The purpose and significance of both our personal and collective endeavours is unearthed.

Through the theoretical and practical content, which includes reading, writing, visualisation, drawing, self-observation, meditation and other exercises, you will learn psychosynthesis at your own pace, thus enabling you to integrate the learning into your daily life. Each chapter focuses on a different aspect of your life journey. The lessons offer you ways to discover more about yourself and increase your self-awareness, thus enabling a more fulfilling life and a clearer connection to your will that can improve your life choices.

To integrate something simply means to combine its parts into a whole, usually in co-operation with someone or something else. Everything we do is integrative. We live not in isolation but with someone or something else—with ourselves, with family, partners, objects, people, the world. This "living with" involves a continual integration—putting together the pieces of ourselves, our relationships to other people, and between ourselves and the world. The process of putting these parts together defines the work of psychosynthesis, always with the aim of co-operating with the process as it naturally happens, thus recognising ourselves as participants within this process rather than its ultimate destination.

While updating psychosynthesis to incorporate contemporary insights is pivotal, it is equally vital to honour its intrinsic vision, especially in recognising that the dark side of our nature is equally part of our life journey as much as the light. By delving into the present's relational intricacies, unearthing the significance of past events, deciphering unconscious messages through dreams and language, and honouring our spiritual depths, psychosynthesis propels us to embrace a deep and wide mindfulness that includes our bodies and the external world.

Psychosynthesis clearly has social as well as therapeutic and spiritual aspects. Nurturing a deeper connection with our divine core intensifies our ability to shed light in our surroundings, transform our environment, and live with spiritual connection. We create the world in which we live through our imagination; our will, properly tempered by love, is the force by which we maintain it.

As we align our personal will with transpersonal purpose (or "true will"), we then have, as Roberto Assagioli, the founder of psychosynthesis expressed it, the strength and the power to express compassion according to wisdom, and the wisdom and compassion to use power for the greatest good.

Studying and applying psychosynthesis in your life is a journey of profound self-discovery and holistic growth. Are you ready to explore within yourself both the heights and depths of human psychology and spirituality?

Starting the journey

What happens to us, from when we incarnate and are born to when we die, has meaning. Through following the lessons in this book, you will learn to recognise where you are on your own life journey, and explore the meaning and opportunity for you at that time. Starting with an overview of the whole journey of life, sometimes called the journey of individuation, you'll grow a sense of the whole process of development and evolution from the perspective of both your outer personality and your inner sense of self. It is exciting to discover and explore that we are not just personalities but that something else runs through our lives, a deeper presence or knowing. This "something" brings meaning to the journey of life, including all the difficult and dark parts of the journey as well as the light and bright bits.

A useful way to look at life is as a cyclical journey within which we go through many smaller cycles involving change and transition. We'll explore these stages in detail through the lessons, starting with the whole life cycle from birth to death, exploring with each cycle the opening and ending of that life stage. We'll also focus on the significant energetic changes that happen through the times of transition from one cycle to the next.

The first exercise is a reflective meditation. You'll learn more in a later lesson about the many different kinds of meditation used in psychosynthesis. Reflective meditation is simply where you close your eyes, turn your attention inside and reflect upon (think about) whatever the chosen subject is. The trick with reflective meditation is not to allow your thoughts to wander off too far from the central subject or theme of the meditation. It is also important to reflect not just from a place of thinking, but to include intuition, feeling, emotion, and sensation. You will learn more about and become proficient at reflective meditation as the course progresses.

If you have not read the instructions (see p. 5) about how to get the most from the lessons, please do so before continuing. Make sure you have your journal or a notebook ready to make notes afterwards.

> After preparation … Close your eyes and pay attention to your breathing, not trying to breathe in any special way but simply allowing your breath to pass in and out of your body. After a few moments, open your eyes and slowly read the meditation, following any instructions.
>
> Be aware of your life as a journey, from conception to birth to death. Within that journey of life, you make many smaller journeys, for instance the journey of childhood, of adolescence, the journey of partnership, and so on …
>
> [remember to pause to reflect each time you see three dots …]
>
> Reflect now that you are starting the journey of this course, a new journey on which you have embarked. At this point in this journey, near the beginning, what are you feeling? What are you feeling right now? …
>
> What do you think about starting this journey? What thoughts are you having right now? Don't censor or judge, for a while just follow the flow of thoughts about where you are right now …
>
> Now bring your awareness to your body—how does your body feel about doing this? What sensations are you experiencing? What is your body saying to you right now? …
>
> Consider your deeper life journey of which this course is just a part. Where are you on your life journey? Are you coasting along, or is it a time of transition and change? Are you more focused on the old or the new, the past or your potential? Are you feeling tuned into your larger life journey, or maybe feeling distant and disconnected? …
>
> Get a sense of what it is that has brought you to be following this exercise in this course at this time in your life. Perhaps it is not all conscious, just trust what comes to you …
>
> Affirm to yourself the rightness to be here now …
>
> Make some notes about your experience with this reflective meditation …

--- ¶ BREAK ---

Cycles within cycles

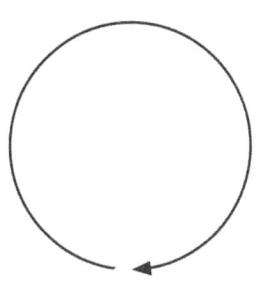

Diagram 1: The cycle of life

Perhaps something happens between death and life, whether something or nothing, no one knows for sure, so we leave a little gap in diagram 1 to show this. Within this whole cycle of life, we go through various other cycles or stages of development. These can be classified in various ways; first we'll consider the seven human ages, based on developmental theories. These are: baby/infant, toddler, child, adolescent, young adult, mature adult and elder (diagram 2).

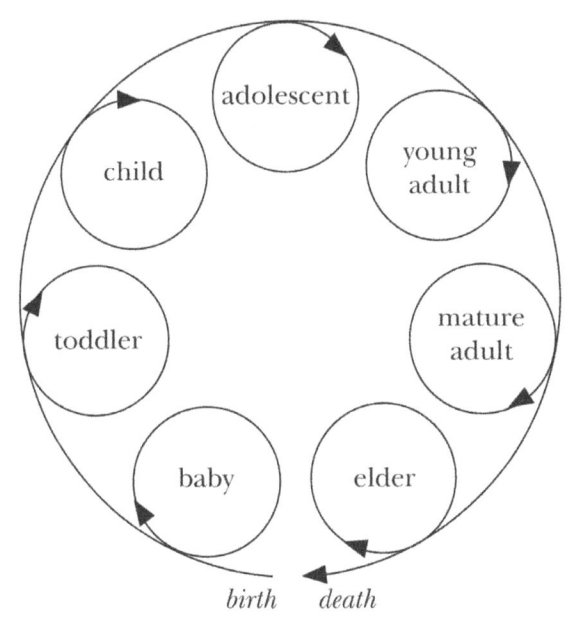

Diagram 2: The seven stages of development

We all go through transitions that take us from one of these life stages to another. For instance, when a baby turns over and starts crawling, they enter the toddler stage; when a child reaches puberty, they enter adolescence. Each passage and each stage have their own signs, symptoms, and peculiarities, which we will be exploring in more detail in future lessons.

Of course, within each of these smaller cycles, there are yet smaller cycles of transition and change. For instance, as you are an adult (I expect!), one of the smaller cycles you are currently engaged in involves your desire to learn and develop. You wouldn't be doing the course in this book if this was not the case. This desire has led you to an interest in psychosynthesis, and then to this course. And here you are today, at this particular time, involved in reading this first lesson (diagram 3).

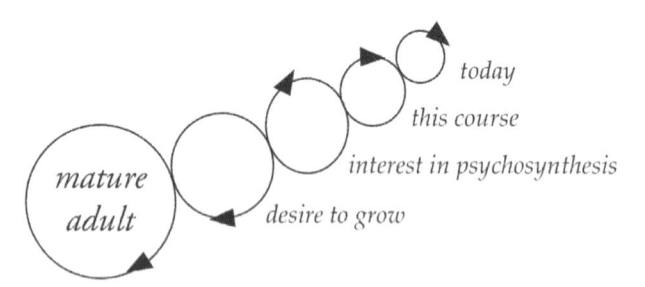

Diagram 3: Cycles within cycles

Another cycle you may be involved in as an adult is that of being a partner to someone. Another cycle in your life journey might involve living on your own. You may have children and are involved in the cycle of parenthood, guiding other beings through their early cycles of development. Within the cycle of parenthood, you might have a difficult adolescent living with you at this moment; and so on.

Part of the value of using this model for life is that it helps us to recognise how feelings, emotions, reactions, thoughts, and many other responses to any situation, instant or ongoing, are patterns that repeat themselves through many of life's cycles. These repeating patterns usually originate in the earlier cycles within your life journey.

> Where are you now on your life journey? ...
> What patterns are you repeating by engaging in this course? ...

And what patterns are you changing? ...
What patterns are you hoping to change by engaging in this course? ... [write]

As you study this model of the cycles within cycles of life and the patterns of behaviour that are constantly being repeated, it is also important to remember the basic, universal truth: that everything changes.

——————————— ¶ BREAK ———————————

Who is here?

It is a good idea when studying, especially when reading, to take regular breaks. Not only does this allow you to relax, taking a break also gives your mind time to assimilate new information and experiences before moving on to what comes next. The following exercise is a short and simple way to bring yourself back to yourself and, the more you practise it, the more you experience its usefulness.

After preparation, close your eyes and say: "I am this" to whatever it is you are experiencing ... Keep this up for a little while ...

Now say: "I am more than this" and open your eyes (staying for a while with whatever you experience) ...

Repeat the first statement ("I am this") with eyes open, then the second statement ("I am more than this") and close your eyes ...

Repeat several times, taking your time to really experience whatever comes up for you as you perform this shuttling between eyes open and eyes closed ...

Finish with: eyes open, ask yourself: "Who chooses to open my eyes?" ... close your eyes ... "Who chooses to close my eyes?" ... [write]

The ground of relationship

The American transpersonal psychologist Angeles Arrien spent several years researching what were the basic rules in indigenous and ancient societies for behaviour during group meetings. Behind the rules are four basic principles that are excellent to bring to any relationship, including the one we are starting to build here, the one between you, the explorer, and this course (your guide).

These basic principles are:

1) show up
2) speak your truth without fear of judgement
3) listen to what has heart and meaning
4) be open to outcome, not attached to it

These are important and also difficult principles to maintain during any relationship, and it is more than likely that you will sometimes not meet up to their demands. If you hold them as the ground on which to build a relationship, however, they offer a solid foundation for all kinds of relationships.

<u>To show up</u> might not be as easy as it first sounds: to maintain your work during this course will require will and awareness, application and imagination. Sometimes issues will arise that you will find difficult to deal with; sometimes inertia and resistance will make it difficult to continue. An important part of the work of learning psychosynthesis is to be able to show up even when it is difficult. Not to force oneself to do something one doesn't want to do, but to bring the difficulties, the resistances and avoidance out into the open and be honest about them. To pretend to yourself that everything runs smoothly if it doesn't, does not serve either you or this learning process.

<u>To speak your truth without fear of judgement</u> is also not easy. We all fear judgements; during early cycles in our life journey, we were subjected to all kinds of conditioning, many different experiences during which we learned to hold ourselves back, or behave in some particular way, as a defence and as a way of survival.

<u>To listen to what has heart and meaning</u> requires trust, and you already have some trust here otherwise you wouldn't have started this course. Nothing is perfect, however, and sometimes the direction might be off the mark, maybe suggest things that don't quite meet your needs. Trust in your own perceptions, feelings, intuition, and insight; your own heart knows what has meaning for you. Part of the work of this course involves being more in touch with and able to build a relationship with your heart so that you recognise what has value in your life journey.

We all have expectations, wishes, desires, some out in the open, some more dark and hidden (even from ourselves). <u>To be open to outcome,</u>

not attached to it is therefore another difficult task. The more you are able to hold this principle in your work, the more you will be in the moment, not prey to past conditioning or future fears and fantasies.

---¶ BREAK---

An autobiographical exercise

Write notes for an autobiographical account of your life to date under the headings: birth, babyhood, toddler, child, adolescent, young adult, mature adult, elder. Don't in any way attempt to be complete but focus on what for you are the main events during these various stages or at the transitions between stages. What is important now is deepening your sense of life as a journey. You can always return to this autobiography again to fill in more detail at another time. You can spend as long as you like on this but an hour or two should suffice for now not necessarily all at once.

Some students find it preferable to create a pictorial representation of their life journey rather than using words, and if that appeals to you that's fine.

When you have finished your writing (or drawing), spend some little while recording in your journal or notepad how this experience was for you, and any responses or reactions you had to creating the autobiography … [write]

Please do not share your autobiography, at least for now. It is confidential and it is important you have it with you for future work.

---¶ BREAK---

An organic process

Psychosynthesis is not only a method for self-realisation, but is a continuous and organic process that is happening in the psyche of everyone at all times. This process happens naturally, but it tends to get blocked. The methods of psychosynthesis include techniques for unblocking this process. These techniques are not used mechanically, but are applied with care and attention. They can then act as transforming agents in our lives, and put us in touch with the natural flow of growth and development.

To help understand the process of psychosynthesis, it has been found useful to split it into two parts: "personal" and "transpersonal" (or "spiritual") psychosynthesis. Personal psychosynthesis concentrates on building a personality that is effective and relatively free from blocks of any kind, is able to direct its energies constructively, and has a clear awareness of its own centre or "I". Central to psychosynthesis is the idea that each of us has a core "self" which, when contacted, helps us organise, and ultimately synthesise, all the various parts that make us up. To reach this centre we have to use our will. This will is not at all like the old-fashioned concept of will power—something that you have to struggle with in order to make things work—but is rather something fluid and easy, something which, as we approach our self or centre, we find becomes easier, and is even fun.

To really harmonise all the various parts of the individual, it is essential to contact this core self, called the "I" in psychosynthesis, around which the synthesis can take place. The more the sense of this "I" is realised, and the more contact is made with it, the more we can then realise our even deeper connection with the transpersonal or spiritual realms. In psychosynthesis this deeper centre is called the Self (with a capital "S" to distinguish it from the self with a small "s", which is another name for the "I"). Don't worry if this seems confusing, it won't be once you experience it.

The first stage of psychosynthesis is, therefore, analysis which helps you get a thorough knowledge of your personality. Next comes the work of personal psychosynthesis, focusing on ways to control and integrate the various parts of the personality. This is based on the main principle of psychosynthesis, which states that we are controlled by everything with which we become identified or attached. We can make choices about everything from which we disidentify or dis-attach ourselves. The first five lessons focus primarily on this personal work, which gives a good ground on which to build deeper exploration of the transpersonal and spiritual realms.

You achieve this shift in your focus through contacting your unique and unattached core self. When you feel the surge of an overwhelming wave of anger, for example, you no longer either need to suppress it or let it take you over and explode out in whatever form it chooses—both ways in which it has you rather than you having it. Instead, you can have the anger and find ways to express it appropriately, or to discharge the energy in other ways (for example, in creative acts) if the anger is inappropriate.

When you have it rather than it having you, the "you" that has it can then say "I have anger (or whatever it is)." Who is this "I" that has it? It is the "I" that is your centre or self, the you that is simply awareness, unattached to anything but willing to identify with the contents of your consciousness as appropriate. Once you have made good strong connections with the "I", the next step of psychosynthesis is the re-forming of your personality around this centre.

Transpersonal psychosynthesis explores the spiritual regions, areas beyond our ordinary awareness. It is in such areas that we find the source of intuition and our sense of value and meaning in life. For many people personal psychosynthesis is enough, as it helps them become harmonious individuals, well-adjusted within themselves and within the communities or groups to which they belong. However worthy an achievement this may be, however, for some people it is not enough and they touch on a real need inside to develop spiritually as well—this is when transpersonal psychosynthesis comes into its own.

Using psychosynthesis we can learn to grow on all levels. We can develop as a personality and find more effective ways to experience life and to express ourselves. We can also grow in our connection to the transpersonal realms, thus unleashing more positive, beneficial qualities into our lives. We find more effective ways of utilising our creative energies. Creativity, in the psychosynthesis sense, is not just about drawing, painting, making music, sculpting or whatever (although it is these things as well), but acknowledges that we are all creative in our own ways. With the right attitude we can be as equally creative doing housework as in painting a masterpiece, in changing a baby's nappy as in encouraging the baby to walk and talk.

Everything in nature appears to be evolving towards increased wholeness. This could even be considered to be the definition of evolution. Psychosynthesis co-operates with this process. An atom comes together with other atoms to form a molecule, and these form cells, which then group into tissues that become organs that make up a whole body. A similar process of synthesis can be seen in our psychological world, too, as all the parts of us come together to make us into one, whole person. We can use psychosynthesis to help us explore all these parts so we become more centred and able to function more effectively. If one molecule was at war with another, and your heart didn't agree with your lungs, you'd have problems. So it is with the psychological functions too—when our sensations, feelings, thoughts, emotions, imagination, intuition, everything that makes us up, are harmoniously synthesised, then we work well and without conflict.

For a true synthesis, the individuality of each part must be respected. No bit of us is "better" or "worse" than another bit. On the contrary, each part has to be whole before it can truly be synthesised and integrated. The conflicts we experience can be seen in this light—as the source of the energy that allows us to know more about ourselves. When we work on our inner conflicts, we can utilise the released energy to bring ourselves through into more effective functioning. In other words, apparent obstacles can be seen as gifts that we can value as much as the more obvious gifts when things are going well.

We can know what we want, and have an idea of where we are going in life, but once we start moving in that direction, we find there are all kinds of blocks that stop us. If we see these blocks as our helpers, then through looking at them and dealing with them, we can more effectively move in the direction in which we desire to go. The blocks are, indeed, the very energy of our being, so the more we deal with the blocks, the more we are moving towards our true being, rather than cutting off from ourselves and not allowing our potential to grow and blossom.

When we start making choices about where we are going or what we want in life, one of the first major obstacles we meet is all the conditioning we have received as children (and often are still receiving through advertising and political control). This conditioning is most clearly seen in the things we believe we "should" do—should go to bed early, should wash your teeth, should be a good girl, and so on. We have to move towards a freedom of choice and not allow these "shoulds" to control our actions. This is not always so easy. We know we "should" do something even though it is not what we really want to do, so how do we do what we want to do without being in conflict with the part of us that says "you should…"? One of the aims of psychosynthesis is to help you understand that you are always bigger than the dynamic of any such conflict. If you move out of the conflict and connect with the self, from this better vantage point you can make clearer decisions.

When we have peak experiences, times when we feel really connected and "right", when everything around us feels harmonious, and our lives are filled with qualities such as Love, Joy, and Truth, we can make positive affirmations that will expand us and help us to include more of these qualities. But we also have to find ways of manifesting or grounding these energies or they will dissipate into illusion. Psychosynthesis deals both with the connection to these qualities and the ways we can ground them. The work is never a process of "getting rid of" something but is rather aimed at transformation through inclusion. Nothing that exists in the transpersonal realms of the spirit is in conflict, so all qualities can easily co-exist. Yet when they come through to the realm of the actual (that is, the personality) then we find that conflicts do exist. Through honouring the transpersonal qualities and getting more in touch with them, then expressing them clearly, we can bring more harmony to our personality. In other words, we are able to manifest more of our potential.

Although you can go to a psychosynthesis therapist (sometimes called a guide) for individual sessions, or to a psychosynthesis group either for training or group therapy, psychosynthesis is basically a system of self-help. This is not to say that seeing a guide or going to a group does not enrich and often speed up the movement towards wholeness, but the ultimate aim of psychosynthesis, whether you learn about it through a book or go to a guide, is to enable you to do it for yourself. Psychosynthesis does not promise any kind of standard result; how any individual's psychosynthesis unfolds depends upon that person alone. With practice, experience, intelligence, and intuition, however, real and satisfactory results can be achieved.

> Write in your own words what you understand psychosynthesis to be ... [write]

--- ¶ BREAK ---

The part and the whole

> After preparation ... Find a comfortable position, either sitting or lying down, where you are relaxed but alert. Take a few deep breaths and allow yourself to become as calm as possible ...
>
> Imagine a single atom. See the nucleus and the electrons spinning around it. Take some time to really imagine this atom clearly ...

Now imagine this atom combines with another atom, then several more atoms until they form a molecule. Imagine a molecule composed of several atoms ...

Molecules can come together to form cells. Imagine you see this happen, imagine your molecule merging with other molecules and cells forming. Take some time to really reflect on this process ...

Every living thing on our planet is composed of such cells. Your body is made up from an innumerable number of cells that have formed themselves into tissues, organs, blood, bones—everything that makes you what you physically are.

Realise that you are made up from cells. Your unity is dependent upon the harmonious interaction between countless cells, which are in turn dependent upon the synthesis of equally countless numbers of molecules and atoms ...

On a physical level, all these parts come together to make up the whole you. Really connect with how wonderful this is. Realise the same is true for your inner world, too ...

All the parts of you—your thoughts, feelings, emotions, sensations—everything that makes you up, is part of this one, whole being you call myself. Allow yourself to really connect with how wonderful this is, too ... [write]

¶ BREAK

Wholeness and fragmentation

We have come a long way since we started exploring the journey of psychosynthesis at the beginning of this lesson. Psychosynthesis sometimes describes this journey as a journey of re-membering, that is, putting the parts back together. This means finding ways to start integrating the different aspects of your personality, and you will begin working with this in more depth in the following lessons as we go deeper into our investigation. It also means putting together the human and divine aspects of our being. We are all both human and divine, and it is important that we honour both poles of this dynamic. It also means putting together the past (all the old ways of being and behaving that we are holding onto) and our future potential, both what we may become in a positive sense and what we fear for the future (the light and dark aspects of potential). By bringing all this together we can create a synthesis and give meaning to life.

Don't worry about what you remember or not, or what you have learned or not learned at this stage. You connect with psychosynthesis through an osmotic process; it slowly seeps in until one day you go "I've got it." In any case, psychosynthesis is a mystery to be lived, not something to be explained away. Psychosynthesis is about learning to live with a vision that comes from the depths of your being. The journey of life is a quest for the self, for the wholeness that can heal our fragmentation. Wholeness is this sense doesn't mean everything being perfect; it means learning to accept and include all aspects of ourselves, including those we like to show and those parts of us we would rather hide away.

¶ BREAK

Before starting the next lesson

Continue familiarising yourself with psychosynthesis, especially:

- Watch for connections from other sources, whether non-fiction books, novels, films, other art forms and so on, from nature and from everyday life, and consider how they may relate to psychosynthesis.
- Give yourself at least one hour during which time you cannot be interrupted. Spend this time considering your life journey. You may like to reflect on the autobiographical notes you made earlier in this lesson, filling in more details and so forth.
- Looking forward, reflect on what aspects of your activities, or life in general, might benefit from closer attention.

LESSON 2

Models of awareness: understanding our inner world

This lesson delves into the intricate facets of human existence, including all the different parts of us, and starts by providing definitions for some of these components while underscoring the uniqueness of everyone's life journey. The lesson emphasises the pivotal role of significant turning points in shaping one's profound life purpose. The journey of life is likened to a heroic journey that includes phases of integration, disintegration, liminality, and awakening.

You are invited to reflect on your own life transitions, considering how these life crises, turning points in our lives, often reveal aspects of our deepest purpose. The lesson underscores the significance of embracing and learning from both joyous and painful experiences, suggesting that each event, whether perceived as a breakdown or breakthrough, contributes to personal growth.

An imaginative exercise guides you through an evolutionary journey, from being an unformed blob to being a fully upright human, prompting reflection on the qualities and challenges of each stage and exploration of further personal evolution.

An analogy of a mineral's transformation through a series of chemical reactions is employed to underscore that personal growth is a co-creative process that impacts both the self and the world.

After introducing and exploring the principal psychosynthesis "map", the "egg diagram", the lesson ends with a focus on taking the next step in your life journey, with self-assessment, goal setting, and an exploration of necessary changes.

Defining who we are

Body, emotions, feelings, thoughts, intuition, soul, and self are the "parts" of us that constitute the person we believe ourselves to be and with which we explore the world around us. Here are some definitions for you to reflect on:

- Body, in the fullest sense of the word, includes everything you experience inside your body, all your sensing, feeling, and thinking (because they all happen inside the body). It is also the physical structure (the "corpse"), which is animated by the "soma" (or "soul"), the living, breathing, energy that you are, and with which you bring your body to life.
- Intuition is a link between body and soul.
- Soul is that part of you that inhabits your body, emotions, feelings, and thoughts and is experienced as your deepest sense of who you are.
- Self is that part of you that is beyond all of this—body, feelings, thoughts, everything you know yourself to be as a personality. In fact, it is more accurate to say that you are part of the Self rather than the Self is a part of you.

> Imagine you have been commissioned to write entries for a dictionary. Research other definitions of the words body, soul, and self, then write your definitions of these words ... [write]

―――――――――――― ¶ BREAK ――――――――――――

Turning points

The whole journey of life is unique to each individual. Beginning with incarnation (or conception), and then from the time of the first cells dividing in the embryo, the journey is one of differentiation.

At times, we experience the focus of our life journey is on integrating our experiences, and there are times when we seem to be disintegrating. In whatever ways we experience all the different aspects of life, we are all affected all the time by what has happened to us in our individual and collective past. We are not victims of the past, however, as throughout life we are sowing seeds that give us clues to our deeper life purpose. We may also experience a deeper sense of purpose, or at least get a glimmer of it, at times of special awakenings, times that are often experienced as life crises.

This journey of life, with both its easier and its more difficult phases, has been described as a hero's journey. Of course, in reality while we may sometimes experience ourselves as heroic, sometimes we experience ourselves as something other than that! Those willing to deeply explore their life journey, however, are offered the ultimate challenge—and rewards—of becoming oneself in the widest and deepest sense.

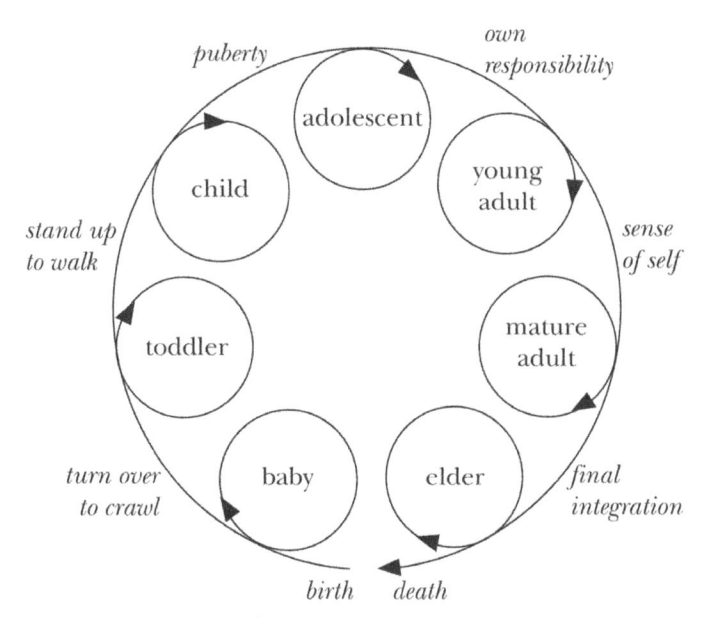

Diagram 4: Transitions on the journey

Spend a while studying diagram 4, which has the same cycles as previously shown but this time paying particular attention to the turning points in a life journey—standing up to walk, puberty, leaving home, and so on.

> After preparation ... Look back once more over your life and get a sense of the journey you are on ... Reflect on the notion that the journey of life is also that of your soul ...
>
> Starting with this week, consider events further back in your life, and as you do so allow times that have been important to you or significant in your life in some way to particularly stand out ...
>
> Consider: What have the crises in your life been like? ...
>
> Consider: Are there significant turning points that you feel brought you back on course regarding your life purpose? ... [write]
>
> Ask yourself: What am I living my life for? ... [write]

---------- ¶ BREAK ----------

Crisis and opportunity

The turning points in our lives could just as easily be called growing points, whether we experience them as growing up or growing down! We grow through both times of joy and times of pain. It has been said that a breakdown can always be reframed as a breakthrough. While in one sense these might be fanciful ideas, in another sense they hold true, especially when we look deeper into the meaning and purpose of these experiences. Our aim is to learn to face suffering with an acceptance, not of a passive kind or as being a victim, but where the acceptance (or surrender) allows us, somewhat paradoxically, to make better choices for ourselves.

Turning points are times when the will is activated, and through learning the lessons presented to us during these times, we bring greater perspective and proportion into our lives. Indeed, perhaps all our experiences of change are part of a larger evolutionary pattern beyond our individual existence. Try the next exercise, which involves a process of evolution.

> After preparation ... Imagine yourself as nothing more than an unformed blob. You have no parts, no edges, no purpose, you simply blob. (You might like to use your body, moving yourself into a position where you feel like a blob.) ...
>
> Now imagine you become a one-celled amoeba ... then a two-celled animal ... then a flatworm ... really imagine what it is like to

be such simple creatures ... You move towards light and food, and away from things that might harm you, but apart from that you are not very conscious. Yet all the while, from being a single-celled amoeba to being a flatworm, you have been becoming more differentiated. In your evolution there has been progress from random wiggling to purposeful wriggling ...

No longer a flatworm, you find yourself moving up the evolutionary ladder, evolving (at least from a human perspective) from being a creature that flops about on its belly to one that has a sense of where it is going, a sense of purposeful crawling. Imagine yourself now evolving from crawling to four-footedness. Imagine yourself as an animal on all fours ...

Really let your imagination run free: what sort of four-footed animal are you? If you feel able, get on all fours and act as if you are this animal, moving round your room exploring your space ...

Now you take the next evolutionary step to become an upright creature, a biped. Imagine yourself going through this process, becoming perhaps an ape, a gorilla, a monkey-like creature of some kind ...

Slowly you move from hesitation to surety. Be aware of changes involved to now move towards the human form. Stand up and be a human, in a human body ...

Now you are fully upright, you have more freedom to express yourself and experience the world. At the same time, you become more vulnerable with the increased openness of your soft underbelly ... How does this feel to you? ...

Be aware of the qualities inherent in two-footed life, including the advantages and the disadvantages. How is it for you to be a human? ...

What is the next step you can now imagine in the evolution of the creature that started off as a blob, became an amoeba, and went through various stages to become a human? Where do you go from here? ...

Use your body to explore this as much as you feel able ...

How can you take on qualities of being human such as, for instance, freedom, refinement, and co-operation? ... [write]

Consider whether there is perhaps something that remains unchanged, right through this whole evolutionary process. For instance, a single

atom of copper (Cu) might combine with some oxygen to become a completely different substance—copper oxide (CuO). The form, properties, and potential of copper oxide are very different from the original copper. This copper oxide then might combine with sulphur to become copper sulphate ($CuSO_4$), which again has a different appearance and properties. Then (perhaps through the application of great heat) the copper sulphate is reduced to its components: copper, sulphur, and oxygen. Is this copper (Cu) the same as the original copper, or has it been changed by its experiences?

In a purely chemical sense it is the same, yet we all know, or feel, or sense, or intuit in some way or another that it is different. From your experience, do you sense this is a good analogy for the evolution of an individual human being?

It is said that the most useful way to view the personality is as an ally that co-operates with the process of the evolution of both the self and the world. The whole process of evolution, from a psychosynthesis viewpoint, is then one of co-creation. What we do affects our world and equally what happens in our world affects us.

---¶ BREAK---

The egg of being

When we are exploring ourselves and our relationship with other people and the world around us, it is very helpful if we have a map. There are lots of different maps of consciousness, some better than others. One of the best maps used in psychosynthesis is sometimes called the "egg of being" or quite simply "the egg diagram".

As you read about the egg diagram, draw it yourself and label the different areas (see diagram 5).

The egg diagram represents the whole psyche. The three horizontal divisions of the egg stand for our past (1), present (2), and future (3). All three are constantly active within us, although in different ways. This is obvious when we consider the present moment—after all, we are here and now, not then and there! Within this present moment, this "here and now", we carry the past with us in the form of all our memories and experiences, whether we remember them or not. It is everything from the past, in one sense, that makes us what we are in the present moment.

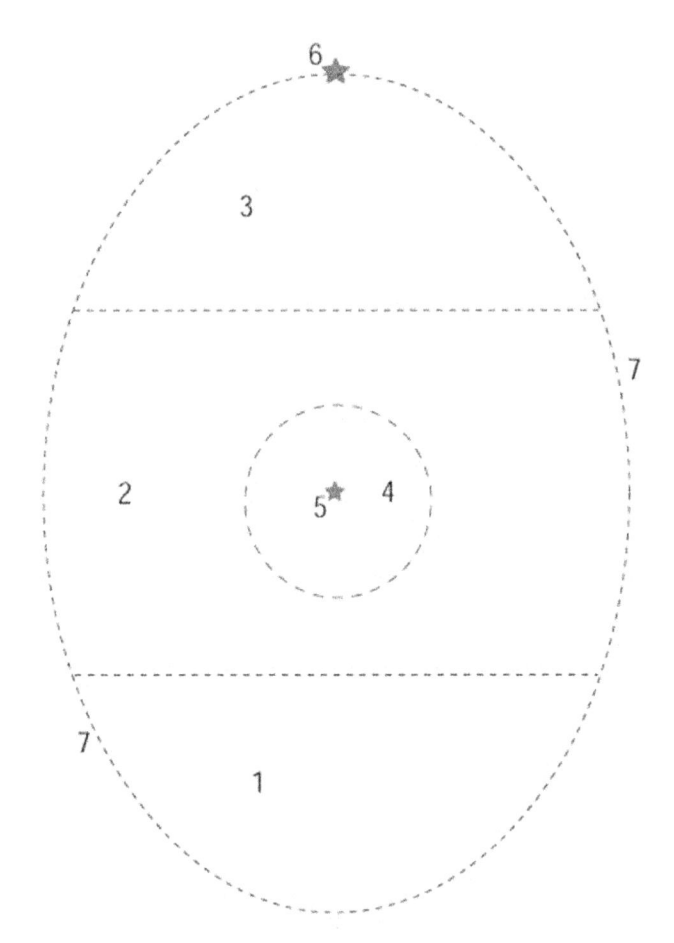

Diagram 5: The psychosynthesis egg diagram

In another sense, perhaps more "esoteric" but no less real, we also carry the future within us. It has not happened yet, but all of us have right now the potential to become something else, to have new experiences, to find new ways to express ourselves. Or perhaps someone's potential might be to always remain the same, to experience or express nothing new—but that, too, is a potential they carry within themselves.

If we look at the egg diagram in this way, we can see it is a complete map of the continuum of time. While its primary focus is on the present moment, because that is, after all, the moment in which we want to use the map, like all good maps it will help us tune into where we have been (the past) and where we are going (the future). By reference to the past, we can get a clearer understanding of where we are in the present moment. This then helps us decide where we want to go and how to get there.

The egg diagram is chiefly concerned, however, with our inner journey, and so its "divisions" represent the different aspects of ourselves as individual beings, and our connection to other beings too. Study the map as you read the following descriptions so that, as your familiarity with the map increases, so does your familiarity with the different aspects of yourself. Even if you have viewed this map before, give it time now—you will learn something new.

(1) represents the lower unconscious, our personal psychological past. This includes repressed complexes, long-forgotten memories, instincts and physical functions over which we (ordinarily) have no conscious control. All our fundamental drives and "primitive urges" are part of this realm as are the activities of basic bodily functions. It is primarily the repressed material, often experienced in the form of unconscious controls upon us, phobias, obsessions, compulsive urges and so on, with which we are primarily concerned in psychosynthesis.

If you had recently travelled through, say a foreign country, all the experiences you would have had would have changed you, and would "colour" your experience right now. Some things might have happened to you that you have pushed out of your consciousness because they are too unpleasant to remember (equivalent to repressed material). Although you might have chosen to "consciously forget" these incidents, they would nevertheless have an effect on you. If you had been chased by a pack of growling dogs, for example, and you only escaped by the skin of your teeth, you might not want to remember their glaring eyes and dripping fangs. Their effect would still be there, however, as shown by your reaction right now to that friendly little poodle!

You might have had it instilled in you as a child that you must wash your hands every time after using the toilet. This in itself is sound advice, but you were conditioned into believing you have to do this or you are naughty. But while travelling, you cannot always do this, and after every time you use the toilet you keep feeling a little sick. Of course, it may be that you are being affected by some bacterium. It could equally be that, although you have forgotten it, you are really being affected by the parental voice that somewhere in your unconscious still tells you off when you don't do what you are told.

These are just two examples of items within us that may affect us at any moment. See if you can think of other such examples, but don't be surprised if you find it difficult—after all, part of the power of such things from the past is that they are no longer remembered and thus exert a much stronger hold on us.

When we explore our lower unconscious, it helps our growth because as we learn to integrate more of these "older" or repressed aspects of ourselves, the more whole we become. When we engage and release previously repressed energies, we feel healthier, have more energy available to us, and feel more freedom in our lives.

(2) represents the middle unconscious, the place where all states of mind reside, which can easily be brought into our field of awareness (4). For example, in our readily accessible "middle unconscious", we carry all sorts of information and knowledge that is not always relevant. We know how to do simple arithmetic, but do we really want to choose to have that in our consciousness when we are making love? We know how to bake a cake, but do we want to be thinking about that when we are reading these pages? You might know that later tonight you have an important meeting with a friend, but you can safely let that knowledge reside in your middle unconscious until later. Of course, if it is a very exciting meeting, then all through the day it will keep popping into your mind, perhaps distracting you from whatever else you are doing.

The middle unconscious also holds suppressed material. This differs from repressed material that has been "pushed down" into the lower unconscious. With repressed things we no longer remember or own them as part of us. Suppressed material, on the other hand, we know is there, it is just that we are choosing, for one reason or another, not to bring it out at this moment. For example, you really want to eat something, but you have to suppress the desire until lunchtime when you are free to go to a café. Or you know something about a friend of yours but you are choosing to suppress this knowledge for fear of upsetting or hurting them.

There is nothing wrong with suppression, but we have to be careful that things that we suppress in our consciousness do not get completely forgotten, and then become part of the contents of our lower unconscious from where they will start controlling us rather than us controlling them.

The field of awareness (or consciousness) (4) is usually shown simply as a circle, but I prefer to imagine it like an amoeba to emphasise how it constantly changes. The field of awareness is constantly alive with sensations, images, thoughts, emotions, feelings, desires and impulses, all of which we can observe and act upon or not as we see fit. One moment you are relaxing with your lover, say, and have a "pseudopod" stretched out to your feelings. Then the phone rings. It is a call from your work, and now you retract the pseudopod that was into feelings, and "stretch yourself", as it were, into a mental place, where you can connect with the conversation about work.

Our field of awareness is constantly fluid, changing as our feelings or thoughts or sensations send us information about our environment. If we become really cut off from our experiences it can be as if the amoeba of awareness "encysts"—it hardens its semi-permeable skin and stops letting through clear messages, either from inside to outside or vice versa. Part of the work of this course is to bring freedom of movement to our amoeba, and to increase our awareness of its function and abilities.

(3) represents the superconscious, our evolutionary future, the region from where we receive all inspiration and illumination, however we experience it. Indeed, true inspiration can come to us in artistic or scientific, very grand or very simple ways. It is the source of our "inner genius", and is thus perhaps the major area of exploration for us when we wish to more clearly and successfully move into our future. We will be exploring the realm of the superconscious later.

Perhaps the most obvious way that most people connect with their superconscious is through insights and "inspirational flashes" that just seem to appear in their consciousness. For instance, you might suddenly grasp the solution to a problem that has been bugging you for days or even longer. Or you might suddenly know more about what you want to do with your life after months of feeling uncertain and directionless. Usually such insights, and other similar experiences, show that the superconscious has been contacted.

The exploration of these three realms, the lower, middle and higher unconscious, is one of the main tasks of psychosynthesis. Any distinction between higher (or super) unconscious and lower unconscious is developmental, not moralistic. The lower unconscious is not bad, or in some sense not as good or as important, it is simply earlier in our evolution. It is described as "lower" simply because it is behind us, and forms the foundation of our present awareness. The superconscious is not merely an abstract possibility but a living reality with an existence of its own. Calling it superconscious (or "higher" unconscious) does not mean it is above us or better than us in some way, but is merely meant to describe the sense that as we evolve and move towards it is as if we are raising our consciousness into new experiences. Alternatively, when insights come from this realm of the unconscious, we often get a sense of things "dropping into place".

(7) represents the collective unconscious that is common to all living beings. We are not isolated pieces of individuality, we are not islands, so although at times we may feel isolated and alone, in reality we are part of a collective field in which all other beings play a part. There is a constant and active interchange between us and all other sentient beings, whether we are aware of it or not.

Note how in the egg diagram the lines are dotted to show there are no rigid compartments impeding free interplay between all these "levels". If we become too rigid it is as if the egg "hardens", and our work might be to crack it a little to let more fluidity into our lives. On the other hand, if we are too sloppy, too "nice" for our own good, if we find it difficult to separate ourselves from other people, then it is as if the spaces in the egg have become too large, letting in (or out) too much. Our work is then to strengthen the eggshell, and create more of an individual identity.

(5) is the personal self, our individual "I" (or "self") who experiences all these different states of consciousness. It is the "I" that experiences itself as having thoughts, emotions and sensations. It is not these changing contents of consciousness (thoughts, emotions, sensations, and so on) but is the inner you that experiences these contents. Generally during life, we do not experience this "I" in a very clearly defined way. The more we work on ourselves through psychosynthesis, the more we can start contacting the "I" and making it a living, experienced reality in our consciousness. In one sense we could say on both a psychological but also a physiological level that the more we get in touch with our "I", the healthier or more whole we become.

This personal self is a reflection or spark of the spiritual or transpersonal Self (6) that is both universal and individual. The realisation of this "transpersonal" Self is a sign of spiritual success and achievement. Awareness of the personal self is the primary goal of psychosynthesis, being the place from where we can effectively direct the personality. This leads to a clearer and fuller contact with, and understanding of, the spiritual Self.

In a deeper sense, what we are calling the "personal self", or "I" in the psychosynthesis sense, is the same as often described as the soul.

In whichever ways you define and understand these words, there is no doubt that the work of developing or connecting to the personal self makes our life feel more "soulful".

> Draw, paint and colour the largest possible representation you can make of the psychosynthesis egg diagram and display it prominently in your home.

--- ¶ BREAK ---

The next step

Nothing in life is more important than the next step you take. Whatever your goals or desires, whatever you want to happen, if you wish to walk from here to there, you can only get there by taking steps. Wherever you are on your journey, the next step is the most important for without taking the next step your journey would cease. This may sound very obvious, but at times we all lose the sense of what our next step is, or how to take this step.

> After preparation ... Reflect on what you have learned about the journey of life so far ... Specifically, what have you learned about your own journey? ...
>
> Consider now: Are there choices you need to make in your life journey? What are the next steps in this process? ... [write]
>
> Are there things you need to accept in your life or are there things that need to change? What are next steps in this process? What needs to happen for your life to progress? ...
>
> Now ask yourself: What is my next step in my life journey? How can I allow this process? How can I follow the voice of soul? What do I really need to make this my life, now? ... [write]
>
> Find some way to embody and enact this next step, at least symbolically; it may be a gesture, words, dance, song, whatever suits you ...
>
> As and when appropriate, do it!

--- ¶ BREAK ---

Sensing, feeling, thinking

Our body (and our physical senses), our feelings (and emotions), and our thoughts (both concrete and abstract) are the three basic functions we use to experience the world and to express ourselves. We recognise who we are through our body, our feelings, and our thoughts. Exploring these three functions, how sensing, feeling, and thinking are interrelated within us, and how they interact with the external world, tells us a lot about ourselves.

These three functions are not really that separate and are truly interrelated. If we look for example at our thoughts, then feelings and sensations will be there too. But it is useful to view them separately both to help us understand them and to help us separate ourselves from them.

To effectively develop our personality, we need a good connection with our body, feelings, and thoughts. This connection can be best made through, whatever is happening to us, being able to tell whether it is truly an experience of sensing, feeling or thinking. We can then get a better picture of which of these functions we use most and which tend to be more overlooked in our everyday life. We can discover whether we are more mentally, emotionally or physically identified. This will change for different situations during life, but with most people there is a general tendency to be primarily either thought- or feeling-oriented.

An important theme in psychosynthesis is to raise the energy of the less well-developed parts, rather than reducing the better-developed parts. It is a principle of psychosynthesis that each function must be healed before it can be synthesised with other functions and fully brought into an integrated personality. If you feel you need to develop a more balanced relationship with your emotions, for example, is it appropriate for you to go to that wild party tonight? Depending upon your individual circumstances it may be beneficial or not for you. But through bringing such awareness to play, and asking yourself such questions, you can make clearer decisions rather than just following whims that might lead you off your chosen path of self-discovery.

Another example is a person who wants to develop their mental function but finds it hard to read anything but monthly fashion magazines. While there is nothing wrong with this in itself, this person might do far better choosing to read more mentally stimulating material. Alternatively, mental skills could be applied to the reading of magazines—analysing their contents, looking at what is really being sold in the pages between the ads, and so on. Part of the skill in working on developing and balancing your thoughts, feelings, and body is finding ways to adapt the current situation, whatever it is, to your advantage. How can you use your setting to aid rather than hinder development?

Look at the relationship between your sensing, feeling, and thinking, asking yourself how well they work together in your personality. Then, when a problem arises, you can take the opportunity to find out more about what is happening underneath, what is behind the imbalance. Then you have the opportunity to work on this at a deeper level. And, it must be stressed, in psychosynthesis we never wish to bring any function down to the level of a lesser function. Instead, we always work to elevate a weaker function so that it rises up to the level of a stronger one. If you are strong in feeling and weaker in thinking, then the work will be to develop the thinking function so that it is raised to the level of the feeling function. At the same time, you work on the stronger function by refining its strength.

Most people generally tend to be more attached to either their thoughts or their emotions, and can thus be described as not just oriented towards thoughts or feelings but as being mentally or emotionally identified. Such identification is useful for it allows us to interrelate with the world around us. We will explore this process of identification more in later lessons.

Psychosynthesis uses various techniques to help us get to this deeper level of understanding. These include "time sharing", which means giving all the functions space for expression in your daily life. If you give space to an angry emotional part of you, for instance, it will then not come up inappropriately at other times, but will more readily "time share" with other personality parts. Another powerful technique is "dialoguing", which means encouraging different functions to communicate with one another to see what each has to say, both in terms of what they need but also what they can give. Whenever you experience a conflict between different parts of yourself, you can help by listening to the voices (and needs) of these parts and find ways (literal or symbolic) to fulfil their needs.

> After preparation ... Considering yourself, would you say you are more mentally, emotionally or physically identified (or in what combination do you find these identifications within you?)? Which function predominates—the thinking, feeling or sensing function? ...

Devise a plan so that your less well-developed function(s) can be brought more into balance with your more well-developed function(s) …

Are you able to start putting this into practice? … [write]

---------- ¶ BREAK ----------

Beyond pathology

Many other things, apart from one's own inner development, affect the whole journey of life. Family, education, social media, and television might be considered to be the big four in our current worldwide society. They in turn are influenced by the cultural and collective structures in place at the time of an individual's development. For instance, modern education in our culture generally emphasises the development of thinking, while the education of feelings and body is given much less emphasis, although this has been shifting in recent years.

There is nothing wrong with how we are, and indeed acceptance of how we are allows us the space to change. As stated earlier, what we are looking for is not really balance but alignment, and this is achieved through inclusion, not exclusion. Each part of us has developed (and will continue to develop) but not necessarily equally. For example, a ballet dancer might have a well-developed body but be totally out of touch with her feelings. A brilliant thinker may well be physically underdeveloped.

How we have developed through our formative years does not necessarily have to be seen as something to which we are victims. We each develop as is appropriate for our life journey. We develop what we need. As the psychologist James Hillman has suggested (with his acorn theory), rather than looking for pathology in our past development, we can find the keys to understanding our purpose for incarnation. This means we cannot just ignore painful issues from the past, or try to transcend them in some way, but can include them as indicators of the deeper purpose within.

The more that each of the functions is available to us the better. If a great thinker is underdeveloped in an emotional way, then it behoves them to develop more as a human being, to work at elevating their connections with feelings. If a great singer can hold and express the deepest emotions but doesn't look after their body… and so on.

The sensing, feeling and thinking model is extremely useful, but for completeness it is important to include the fourth function, the intuition. This function is the link between our physical existence and our soul or "source", which is responsible not only for intuition but also for synchronicity and all other ways the Self chooses to reveal itself in our lives.

Intuition

Intuition is very different from "psychic intrusion", and comes when a contact is made between soul and your personality, your "divinity" and your "humanity". To be able to fully and clearly receive intuitions, however, you need to work on your personality so they are received in a harmonious way, with as little distortion as possible. Your receptacle has to be suitable or the messages you receive will be unclear.

When we investigate the functions of the brain, and look at the different modes of thought of which we are capable, we initially see a primary split between abstract and concrete functions. There are no sharp divisions between these two, rather a more gradual division where one merges into the other, but they can, for convenience, be viewed separately. We hear a lot these days about the right and left brain functions (although some recent research suggests this is far too simplistic a model of brain functioning). Whether it is a good description or not in terms of the actual physical organ we call a brain, it is a useful division to help us understand the abstract and concrete thinking modes that we all can experience.

The left brain (connecting to the right side of the body) is concerned with rational and linear modes of operation. From the left brain you think, order, make lists and organise your life and actions. It is from here that concrete thinking takes place. The right brain (connecting to the left side of the body) is concerned with non-rational, intuitive, non-linear modes of operation. From the right brain you feel, intuit, make crazy connections, and generally live in a non-ordered, more fluid way. Both sides are of equal importance and both are equally necessary for the full and healthy functioning of the individual. Problems only arise when one assumes an unhealthy dominance over the other, or there is a critical identification with one or other of the ways of operating.

Concrete functions (left brain, thinking and sensing) involve physical matters; they help us to understand our actual, physical existence, our functioning here on planet earth, in this dense earthy energy.

Abstract functions (right brain, intuiting and feeling) involve making connections in a non-linear, non-verbal way, helping to increase our awareness and process our expression of who we really are.

We are all moving towards greater awareness. Anything abstract, or non-manifest, can come to life through a number of forms. It can emerge through your thoughts, feelings or body, perhaps as a "sense" or "feeling" or "flash" of knowledge and understanding. Patterns are trying to emerge, and the more we are open to their emergence, without trying to force them into a particular form, the better they are able to emerge. If a triangle is emerging you will receive its wisdom more easily, and more clearly, if you can create a triangular receptor in your being with which to receive it. Fitting squares into round holes is a far more difficult, and daunting proposition. In other words, the more we do to connect with our deeper, innermost nature, and the more we create a well-functioning personality, the better able we are to receive or channel the inner wisdom and unfoldment of purpose that is inevitably trying to emerge into consciousness.

> Reflect for a while on how you could relate the four functions—intuition, thinking, feeling, sensing—to the egg diagram ... [write]

--- ¶ BREAK ---

Summary of influences on our development

Our development is affected by:

- all the events that have happened to us in our lives (the effect of the past, represented in the psychosynthesis egg diagram by the lower unconscious);
- the potential we manifest each time we take the next step on our journey (the middle unconscious);
- the pull we feel within ourselves to know ourselves better as spiritual beings manifesting on this physical plane (the effect of the superconscious upon us).

All this development is directed by the "I" (or "self"), which has a connection to the deepest transpersonal Self. In other words, we are developing body, feelings, and thoughts as vehicles for expression and for the incarnation and manifestation of the deeper Self.

> Spend some while now reflecting on your life journey from the perspective of all you have read so far (maybe an hour or so, maybe a day or two, trust what feels right to you) ...
>
> After some time for allowing this to sink in and deepen, ask yourself:
>
> How do I feel now about my relationship to my body, feelings and thoughts?
>
> What is my attitude towards my body, feelings and thoughts?
>
> Does this attitude need to change and, if so, how? ... [write]
>
> What simple act, real or symbolic, could you find to start to express this in the world?

¶ BREAK

Global awareness meditation

Later in the course we will be exploring how the psychosynthesis approach can help us find our way in the confusing, tumultuous experience of being alive in the modern world. How we respond to all the news of global events—of a positive or negative nature—affects us deeply.

> After preparation ... Reflect on a major world issue, either local or distant. Pick one, and consider what you know about it, feel about it, and sense about it ... [write]
>
> Turn your attention inside and consider the issue you chose for your reflection. How did you choose it? ... Why did you choose it? ... Who chose it? ...
>
> How do you feel about it now? ...
>
> What does what you picked reflect of you, or say about you? ...
>
> In what ways do you project yourself into this problem? ...
>
> In what ways do you negate or ignore your response to this problem? ...

Now sit quietly and reflect on the question: "who am I?" Each time you ask yourself this question, as an answer comes, write it down. Don't judge or censor or try to interpret what answers come, trust in your own inner responses … [write]

---------------- ¶ BREAK ----------------

Before starting the next lesson

Continue familiarising yourself with psychosynthesis, especially:

- Watch for connections from other sources, whether non-fiction books, novels, films, other art forms and so on, from nature and from everyday life, and consider how they may relate to psychosynthesis.
- Give yourself at least one hour during which time you cannot be interrupted. Spend this time considering your relationship with your body, sensations, feelings, and thoughts. You may like to use your autobiographical notes to see how this relationship has changed (or not) over the years.

LESSON 3

Subpersonalities and self-expression: exploring our many roles

In this lesson we start to explore the concept of subpersonalities, which are the various aspects and roles of your personality. Different subpersonalities can have conflicting desires and needs, and the lesson encourages self-reflection for you to explore and identify your own subpersonalities. It emphasises that recognising and owning these subpersonalities can lead to a more harmonious and unified whole personality.

A major aspect of subpersonality work is discovering the wants and needs of each, and differentiating between them. Subpersonalities have conflicting wants, and understanding their underlying needs can help resolve these conflicts. This is followed up by exploration of the archetypal energies of Love and Will and how they can manifest through subpersonalities. The importance of unifying these energies is highlighted, as is the potential for personal growth and transformation through self-awareness and integration.

The lesson concludes by asking you to reflect on your progress in understanding your subpersonalities and their relationship with different aspects of yourself. It also prompts you to consider the qualities that each subpersonality represents, and how to integrate and express these qualities in your life.

Review

Did you give yourself at least one uninterrupted hour considering your relationship with your body, sensations, feelings and thoughts?

If not, reflect (and write) on your reasons for this. This is not about making judgements on yourself, or you being judged in any way, but to help you to uncover more of the workings of your psyche.

Seen and not seen

Life often seems to be an endless struggle between different parts of us wanting different things. The more we look at ourselves, the more it seems we are not whole, but composed of lots of different parts all having their own needs and desires. We are not split personalities but rather multiple personalities. Each of the "little personalities" within us is called, in psychosynthesis, a subpersonality. Each subpersonality has a part to play in our lives and we all play many parts, often with conflicting thoughts and feelings about what is good for us, or even of who we actually are.

You might be a "mother" seeing your children off to school, then the very next minute a "housewife" washing the dishes. Later that morning you are a "dancer" in your Pilates class, then a "friend" for someone over lunch. Meanwhile your "husband" has become a "businessman" in his office. Later tonight you will be alone together and become "lovers".

All of us play such roles, often apparently flitting from one to another part with consummate ease. Yet how conscious are we of these parts we play? Do you easily slip into a part of yourself that blushes and feels shy when in a crowd? Do you become an angry part of yourself just because you missed a bus? Are there times when you get "stuck" as a housewife or a banker and wish things could change? Or perhaps you are so identified with a role you do not even realise it is a role you are playing. Instead, you think it is the "real" you.

How we like to be seen, by others and by ourselves, and what parts or aspects of ourselves we hide away (from others and from ourselves!) are useful starting points for a deeper exploration of subpersonalities.

> After preparation ... Reflect on: How do I like to be seen? What is it I like others to see in me? What parts and aspects of myself do I like to show? What constitutes the acceptable me? ...

Now consider: What are the behaviours that go with all this? How do I behave so people see me the way I want? And when did these behaviours start—how old was I? Who else was involved? and so on ... [write]

As a result of these behaviour patterns that you've just been reflecting upon being set up, there were aspects and parts of yourself that you were unable to show (for fear of being unacceptable in some way or another). Consider: As a result of these behaviour patterns being set up, what aspects of myself was I not able to show? ...

Do these aspects of myself still operate now? ... [write]

Reflect on the relationship between the two aspects of yourself (what you show and what you don't show). What is their attitude to one another? Are they on speaking terms? If so, what is the dialogue between them like? ... [write]

We'll look more deeply into these parts later, but for now it is certainly time for a break.

─────────────── ¶ BREAK ───────────────

The multiple personality

One good analogy for our personality is seeing it as like an orchestra. Then all these different parts or roles we play are like the members of that orchestra. As we become more able to define our lives, and control our processes in a positive inclusive way, we become like the conductor, allowing each individual member to play a part, and working towards orchestrating the personality into a harmonious whole.

This conductor is the self or "I". As the conductor we will also contact the composer, the transpersonal Self, who will supply us with information about how to play the musical composition of life and also, perhaps, information about each individual player's part in the whole. In Lesson Six you'll explore these "executive features" in depth and learn how to self-identify (that is, become the "conductor" of your inner orchestra). First, though, it is important to thoroughly explore your subpersonalities in detail.

One way to start learning more about our different subpersonalities is to give them names. Roberto Assagioli suggested naming each of our subpersonalities with humour, both as a way of connecting to their energies but also to maintain a healthy detachment and "lightness" in this work. So, for example, a rather crazy emotional part of your personality could be called "Crazy Chris"; a bossy part "Mrs Knowitall"; a rather dreamy little girl "Alice" (in Wonderland); and so on. By giving our subpersonalities such names, we have identified them as not being all that we are, and have given them a handle by means of which we can interact with them.

Spend some time now thinking about your different subpersonalities. It is a good idea to make a list of the main ones, then see how many you can name. Thinking of your more prominent traits, attitudes and motives will help you start. For each part of you let an image emerge. It may be the image of a human of any gender, or an animal, a mythical creature, or anything at all. Do not make up these images for your subpersonalities, but rather let them spontaneously emerge from your unconscious.

You can start with the more obvious roles such as husband or wife, partner, daughter or son, businessperson, sportsperson and so on. Take care, though, a role might involve more than one subpersonality. For instance, "Handyman Harry" is a plumber but his role as plumber involves several subpersonalities, for example, the businessman, the trader, the friendly workman, and so on, but also less obvious ones, for instance, a little boy subpersonality who has to have his needs met otherwise he creates problems for Harry, or an "angry raver" who needs his needs met so he doesn't inappropriately explode with anger if things aren't going well.

Then consider subpersonalities that are more based around different states—the miserable old man, the angry cat, the fool, the controller, the top dog, the mystic, the sad little girl, the sensible adult, the shy boy, and so on. The aim is not to have the longest list of subpersonalities in town, but rather to know which subpersonalities you are aware of right now in your life. The list will change, and you can always add more subpersonalities as your work on yourself progresses

> After preparation ... Do what it says: start making a list of your subpersonalities. Write the list as if they are characters in a play, giving each one a name, and a brief description of the image and role of each one ... [write]

¶ BREAK

The difficulty with identifications

When we first think of our subpersonalities, those we most easily connect with are part of what can be called our "core personality". These are subpersonalities we happily include as part of us, included in our sense of who we really are. Some of these will be well integrated and be very helpful to us in our lives. They form the basis of what is sometimes called "the ego" (though be careful, as there are several different ways of using this term). They constitute who we believe we are.

Other subpersonalities are more suppressed. They lie on the boundary between the middle and lower unconscious; we know they are there but we don't happily accept them as part of ourselves. Depending upon the conditioning we have had, and various other developmental factors, they might include subpersonalities that represent "forbidden sexual drives", parts of us that we hide away because we believe them unworthy, powerful parts of us that frighten our sense of who we are. They might also include self-assertive parts, which may become distorted into aggressive subpersonalities. They also include social conditioning, for instance, the "top dog" who is always telling us what to do or not do. For some people, almost everything they do is accompanied by the voice of an inner top dog telling them whether it is "right" or "wrong", whether they should or should not be doing whatever it is. All of these suppressed subpersonalities are often projected onto other people.

Hidden deeper in the lower unconscious are repressed parts of us, primitive parts that are trapped and totally not accepted. They constitute what is sometimes called "the shadow". These parts of us can hardly be called subpersonalities, as we know so little of them. They emerge and control us at times, but generally we keep them well repressed. We have to learn to face these parts of us, so we can release the energy we are using to hold them down. When we release this energy, we usually find we have grown and transformed, perhaps only in a small or subtle way, but nevertheless in a very real and tangible way.

Psychosynthesis aims to expand our consciousness to include all our subpersonalities. We can only transform them when we connect with and fulfil their basic needs. Until then we remain fragmented. A fragmented personality might include a part that split off, as if in trance, acting as if it is "not at home". Cut off from any true, direct experience, if it does express itself, it is often through pleading for its wants in a very unbalanced way. Or we might include a part of us that finds its identity through others, always wants more, never feeling like it has enough. A subpersonality like this only knows where it stands when in relation to someone (or something) else; otherwise, it feels lost, and will generally do anything in its power to avoid these feelings of despair.

We can become so identified with some of the roles we play, it becomes very difficult to let go of them. Imagine a mother whose child has grown up and is ready to leave home. She loves this child and wants the best for them, but she is so attached to the role of mother the separation makes her very sad. She is clinging to her role, and it is only through facing the sadness and accepting the loss that she will release enough energy to be able to move on. When she gets through this, and gives up her old role, she finds she has not "lost" the child at all. And in no longer being so identified with the role she can, paradoxically, play it better.

Or imagine a man who has worked from 9 until 5 in an office for most of his life. He has now retired and, sadly, he has been so identified with his role in his office, he doesn't know what to do with his newfound time and "freedom". He feels bored, at a loss, and even catches himself wishing he could be back at the office. The retirement he has looked forward to no longer seems so attractive. He will have to find very definite ways to let go of his old role, and cultivate new interests to replace the old.

> After preparation ... What is (are) your major identification(s)? ...
> Why is it impossible to fully answer that question? ... [write]

¶ BREAK

Wants and needs

We all know people who, at least in some aspects of their lives, have not "grown up". For example, there might be a 30-year-old man who still plays with his train set—perhaps when he does this, he is really identified with one of his subpersonalities who is still a 10-year-old boy. Perhaps to avoid some of the painful issues he felt in adolescence he reverts, as it were, to an earlier time. Of course, another adult might have a train set for completely different reasons. Or imagine a 50-year-old woman who still acts like an adolescent girl when men are around.

We all have examples of such subpersonalities within us. It is as if all our "little selves" are at different stages of development, some having reached full maturity, others at younger stages, even infantile when confronted with painful or difficult issues.

There is no suggestion that there is anything wrong with having subpersonalities, far from it. They provide us with the means to interact with ourselves, other people and the world in general. Every subpersonality has an important part to play in our total being. Problems arise when they have got you rather than you having them. You come home after a day's work and you cannot stop thinking about it. Yet to "disidentify" from the role you might only need to simply take a bath or shower and put on different clothes.

Psychosynthesis offers us techniques whereby we can discover the roles we play and then more clearly choose to either identify with them when appropriate or disidentify from them when that is appropriate. This way our lives become more harmonious and we are more able to make choices about what we really want. Psychosynthesis, in other words, helps us to both become the conductor of our life orchestra, but also to play all the parts in the orchestra that we wish to play. Yet, even if it were so easy, we can be so caught up with our identifications that we forget ways we may have learned to "shift our awareness".

> After preparation … Reflect on each subpersonality on your list, considering: What does this subpersonality want? and then: What does this subpersonality need?
> [write] answers in your list, to create a table something like:
>
> | NAME | IMAGE | ROLE | WANT | NEED |
> |---|---|---|---|---|
> | e.g. | | | | |
> | Knowitall | Mad prof. | Intellectual | Attention | Recognition of self |
> | Little me | Small child | Connection | Care | Love |
> | Lazy bee | Teenager | Protection | Direction | Purpose |
>
> Be as specific as you can be.
>
> Also be realistic: firstly, accept you may well not be able to recognise the want and need behind each subpersonality; secondly, to not just make it up. To do this exercise effectively, you have to meditate upon the behaviour, wants and needs of each

subpersonality, perhaps create exercises to meet each one in your imaginative world (in the meadow, in a house, garden, etc.), and start to satisfy the genuine needs of that part.

N.B. The aim of this exercise is not to be able to complete it, but to start this work, which can then be an ongoing process of inner exploration. If you feel stuck, or not really connecting with the wants and needs of your subpersonalities, don't worry, feel free to read on and return to work more on your subpersonalities later.

---------- ¶ BREAK ----------

The garden of beauty

In the next exercise you will meet a subpersonality who will take you into a garden of roses. Enjoy the experience of this, and see how subpersonalities are not always in conflict, either with each other or with you. And remember you don't necessarily have to "see" anything; what is important is to get a sense of whatever it is you are being asked to do. Allow your other senses to be present: feel it, sense it. You can very effectively imagine yourself in, as in this case, a rose garden, without actually "seeing" anything.

> After preparation … Taking a few deep breaths. Imagine you are in a meadow, and spend some time tuning into being there. What is the sky like? Is it a sunny day? How do you feel? What can you hear—bird song perhaps? Smell? See? Really be in your meadow, as if it really exists …
>
> In one direction you can see a small house or cottage. Walk that way, feeling your feet on the ground, and remembering to pay attention to being there. As you reach the house, you realise it is the home of some of your subpersonalities. You wonder who will live there, and how they will greet you. As you approach the door be aware of your excitement and anticipation …
>
> You tap, and the door is opened. Greet the person there, and pay attention to what they look like. Is it a man or a woman or a child? Old or young? Fill in as much detail on this figure as you can. Then exchange some words, asking the figure its name if you like. Find out something about this person …

The subpersonality then asks you into the garden. It is a beautiful rose garden. Pay attention to the roses, their colours, scents and overall beauty. Allow yourself to be infused with their quality. Walk with the subpersonality into the depths of the garden, then find one particular rose to which you are attracted.

Both you and the subpersonality look at this rose, brightly lit by a ray of sunshine. Feel the energy, beauty and warmth of the rose transform your feelings and thoughts. Really be whole, feeling good to be there at this time ...

Then turn to the subpersonality and see if it has changed. Engage them in dialogue and ask how they feel, what transformations, if any, may have taken place. Ask particularly about what the subpersonality needs ...

Finally, thank the subpersonality for taking you to the garden, say goodbye for now, and bring your consciousness back to your room.

Write about the experience, and the needs of the subpersonality, in your diary. In what way(s) can you express and fulfil this need, or at least some aspects of it in your daily life? ... [write]

--- ¶ BREAK ---

Beyond conflict

Our subpersonalities know what they want and are determined to get it. They really look out for themselves. This can be all right in itself, but problems arise when what one subpersonality wants is in conflict with the wants of another one. For instance, part of you might want to go to the cinema while a different part of you wants to stay at home. Perhaps one part of you might really need to leave a deadening job but another scared part won't let it happen.

Some of the deepest conflicts can arise between "thinking identified" and "emotionally identified" subpersonalities. You feel like telling someone you love them but you think they will laugh at you. Or you know it is a good idea to take regular exercise but part of you feels too lazy. Such inner conflicts can emerge in rather contradictory ways. A man might be a strong boss at the office but at home a weak husband and father. One day you might go out and be the life and soul of a party, the next you are a mass of nerves, frightened of going out to the corner shop. The work in harmonising the relationship between the thinking and feeling functions can lead to the release of creative energy. This creative energy will be accompanied by the emergence of transpersonal "qualities" such as Love, Joy, Truth and Beauty.

To harmonise the wants of different subpersonalities, it is necessary to get behind them to the deeper level of "needs". Needs are more inclusive than wants: "I want you to kiss me right now" and "I want to respect your own choice" might be conflicting wants. When we contact the underlying need—perhaps "needing more affection in life generally"—then we can find ways to fulfil this need without conflict.

We can make this shift from wanting to needing through simply identifying the initial conflict, then accepting it. We have to accept that if we cannot get away from it, we might as well include it. Once we are able to accept the wants of both sides of the conflict, a transformation is possible.

With all our subpersonalities we need to get to know them. We do this through dialoguing with them, letting them have a voice and realise their wants are being heard. Then we build a true relationship with them in which we attend to the larger needs of all concerned. We can learn to love all our subpersonalities in spite of their faults, and in doing this we give them the space they need in order to grow.

Wants can be harsh and demanding whereas needs tend to be more flexible. Needs are also closer to the essence at the core of the subpersonality. By moving towards this essence, you allow the underlying transpersonal quality to manifest more clearly. This then fuels the transformation towards unification of the personality.

Subpersonalities tend to be either ones who want everything (that affects them) to change, or ones who want everything to stay the same. These wishes usually interact in a dynamic way with the need for love or power. A love-type subpersonality, for instance, might want change: "everything would be better if only you loved me". Another love-type subpersonality might not want change: "I couldn't live without you." Psychosynthesis teaches us to co-operate with the process as much as possible, to choose change when that is most appropriate or to choose stability when that is the better choice.

To reach closer to the transpersonal Self, we have to learn to trust in both things that change and in things that stay the same, and at the same time not be attached to either. Awareness has to be coupled with psychological mastery. We can use our will power to stop us slipping mindlessly into different subpersonalities, but instead to be able to choose, at any moment, the most appropriate role to play. We have the ability to become the driver of our car, not just be a backseat passenger.

The qualities that emanate from transpersonal levels become "degraded" in the personality: trust becomes foolishness, courage becomes foolhardiness, compassion self-pity, and so on. Psychosynthesis helps us realise this, and it also helps us reverse the process. Qualities can also be "elevated" in the personality—our self-pity becoming compassion and so on. The more we work in this way, the less distortions there are in our daily living. Although we might never reach complete unity, the more we move in that direction, the less distortions there are. If we could ever reach total unity in ourselves, we would be free of all conflicts and distortions.

When we do any subpersonality work, it always releases energy, and in so doing allows us to move closer to our centre and our true self. This expresses itself through the increased harmony we then find in our lives. Our multiple personality, our "orchestra", as it grows and harmonises, becomes the ultimate healer of our divisions and fragmentation.

> After preparation ... Continue working on your subpersonality list, including now adding another column to your table: the Quality behind each subpersonality.

NAME	IMAGE	ROLE	WANT	NEED	QUALITY
e.g.					
Little me	Small child	Connection	Care	Love	Compassion
Lazy bee	Teenager	Protection	Direction	Purpose	Will

Remember that it is not always possible to recognise the wants and needs of different subpersonalities, and this applies even more so to locating their qualities. When you are satisfying the genuine needs of each part, you may then really deeply connect with where this energy is coming from.

Needs have been described as the holes through which the Self shines. In that case, qualities are the light itself. Remember the aim of this work is to continue an ongoing process of inner exploration. It must be stressed no hierarchy is being presented here. The process of discovering the behaviours, wants, needs and qualities of a subpersonality is not a linear process. It is not the case that you are a better person because you know all your qualities, or a poor case because you only just barely recognise let alone accept or integrate aspects of yourself. Psychosynthesis is about travelling the path of self-discovery, not about achieving some (probably imagined anyway) goal.

--- ¶ BREAK ---

Subpersonality and other

This next lesson focuses on love and relationship, perhaps the most important and far-reaching topic for any form of study. Everything we do happens in relationship (to ourselves, to other individuals, to groups of people, to other creatures, to trees, rocks... everything in our world!). Use your understanding of your subpersonalities to help you start to explore your "little selves" in relationship with other "little selves".

> After preparation ... Consider: Which of your subpersonalities like to be in relationship? With whom and in what ways? ... [write]
> Which of your subpersonalities do not like to be in relationship? How do they attempt to keep you separated? ... [write]

--- ¶ BREAK ---

Love, will, change and maintenance

The four major archetypes that manifest through subpersonalities are Love, Will, Change and Maintenance. These archetypal energies create the pattern of existence.

Love and Will are the two primary energies that may be in conflict in a personality. They need to be unified. Each subpersonality plays out one of these archetypes—is it content with simply being, does it want to be loved, or does it want to do, to act, perhaps to control? When does it feel sad or hurt? Where does anger come from—your connection to love or your connection to will?

It is important to find out the answers to these questions, but this is done most effectively through the overall process of your work rather than through trying to mentally calculate answers. You have to particularly watch for complex layering of these patterns. A certain part of you may feel angry, so you may think it a distortion of will energy, then you find it is really sad underneath and your orientation changes. Then perhaps underneath that it is angry again.

You can move a love-orientated subpersonality towards unity by including it, listening to its needs, taking care of it. A will-orientated subpersonality is moved towards unity by expressing its needs, directing it clearly, letting it out from its restrictions in a harmonious way.

Of course, these parts have various ways of expressing their "existential belief", and often this is very clear once they are encouraged to express their position. For example, a subpersonality might say: "I won't be loved if I own my own power"; or "I want to be perfect so everyone will love me." Where do these subpersonalities fit into the dynamic of love and will?

It is wonderful how wise our inner processes can be once given the space to expand and integrate. Often, we can see the unfoldment of Will energies through more mentally connected parts of our personality, and of the Love archetype through more emotional parts of ourselves. While this is generally true, however, it is not always the case: the Will can manifest through emotions and Love through the mind. Indeed, in some esoteric systems much is made of this "crossing of the energies", whereby it is said a new, clearer understanding of the relationship between Love and Will can emerge and manifest.

With all subpersonality work, there is no "right" level to reach, and nothing wrong with finding you can go no deeper towards your core. What is important is to honour your own processes and, as your inquiry deepens, to recognise and own what you find underneath the surface layers. That way you are co-operating with the process of your personal evolution.

―――――――――――― ¶ BREAK ――――――――――――

Appraisal

After preparation ... Reflect on how you are doing on this course so far. Check how well you feel you are assimilating the material ...
Write a report on this.

―――――――――――― ¶ BREAK ――――――――――――

Subpersonalities and polarity

In an earlier exercise in this lesson, you were asked to reflect on the relationship between two aspects of yourself (what you show and what you don't show). Consider these two aspects of yourself once more, having your previous notes handy to remind you.

> After preparation ... Reflect on the part of yourself you like to show most ... Allow an image for this part of you, this subpersonality with whom you like to identify. See it standing before you, just to one side ...
>
> Now reflect on a major aspect of yourself you don't show, that you usually hide away ... Allow an image for this part of you, this subpersonality with whom you don't like to identify. See it standing before you, to the other side of the first one ...
>
> Turn back to the first subpersonality and consider how it is dressed, how old it is, what does it look like? What are its typical behaviours? How do you feel towards it? ...
>
> Imagine yourself becoming that subpersonality. What does it feel like to be this part of you? What do you want? What do you need? What do you really need? ...
>
> What would it be like not to get that need met? ... What would it be like to get that need met? ...
>
> What would it be like if you were always only this part of you? ...
>
> What would be missing if this subpersonality was gone? ... What is the value this subpersonality brings to your life? ... [write]
>
> Step back into yourself and shake off that subpersonality ...
>
> Now turn to the second subpersonality. Consider how is it dressed, how old is it, what does it look like? What are its typical behaviours? How do you feel towards it? ...
>
> Imagine yourself becoming that subpersonality. What does it feel like to be this part of you? What do you want? What do you need? What do you really need? ...
>
> What would it be like not to get that need met? ... What would it be like to get that need met? ...
>
> What would it be like if you were always only this part of you? ... What would be missing if this subpersonality was gone? ...

SUBPERSONALITIES AND SELF-EXPRESSION   61

What is the value this subpersonality brings to your life? ... Step back into yourself and shake off that subpersonality ...

Now write about this second subpersonality, and what you discovered about the two parts of yourself from this exercise ... [write]

--- ¶ BREAK ---

A deep reconnection

After preparation ... Reconnect once more to the two subpersonalities you have just been working with. Imagine them on either side of you ... Notice your relationship to them, and how they relate to one another.

Have there been any changes? ...

As you look at both, look deeper into the heart of each subpersonality, to what quality each one of them is trying to express in your life ...

Holding these two qualities, ask yourself: what it my next step:

- in terms of accepting I am different at different times, that I have many faces and that each expresses different aspects of myself?
- and in terms of integrating these two parts of myself more into my life? ... [write]

--- ¶ BREAK ---

Before starting the next lesson

- Continue to reflect on your relationship with your subpersonalities, particularly as they interact with other people. Don't make this judgemental, simply observe the responses and reactions of your subpersonalities to the behaviour of others' subpersonalities, and vice versa.

- What is your favourite novel or story-book? Reflect on how an understanding of subpersonalities might enlighten both your knowledge and your feelings about the characters in this book. Whose subpersonalities are these characters?
- Give yourself at least one hour during which time you cannot be interrupted. Spend this time considering your relationship with your subpersonalities.

LESSON 4

Love and relationship: towards balance and harmony within

Lesson 4 delves into the complexities of human relationships and their impact on personal development. It emphasises the role of early experiences and the projection of unmet needs onto others. The importance of understanding and accepting yourself as you are is stressed as the first step in building healthier relationships.

We explore the mother–child bond, the development of the ego, and the interplay between oneness and separateness. Reflecting on your relationship with your inner self, your parents and others is paramount in releasing true love that can be both selfless and self-sufficient.

A particularly powerful exercise at the end of the lesson promotes a deeper connection with others, encouraging you to see beyond superficial layers to the essence of another person. It also emphasises the importance of choice and maintaining appropriate boundaries in real-world relationships.

Overall, the lesson provides a holistic perspective on relationships and advocates for a conscious and balanced approach to love and understanding.

Review

Did you reflect on how an understanding of subpersonalities might enlighten both your knowledge of and your feelings about the characters in your favourite novel or story-book?

Did you give yourself at least one uninterrupted hour considering your relationship with your subpersonalities? If not, reflect (and write) on your reasons for this. This is not about making judgements on yourself, or you being judged in any way, but to help you to uncover more of the workings of your psyche.

Self in others

Our unmet needs, particularly those of our inner child, which we will specifically explore in more depth in the next lesson, can get projected out in relationships. We see the other (person, creature, group, etc.) through the filter of our expectations. For example, because his mother was unable to meet his need for attention (and not necessarily all the time), a man might project mother on his wife then constantly court her attention. And be angry when he doesn't get it (all the time).

The patterns that are set up in our early relationships, during the time of our "primary scenario", become repetitive patterns through which we live our lives. Then we may find we are living through our fantasies, which are chiefly based upon past successes and failures. The following exercise guides you into finding out more about yourself from how you view others and how they view you, or at least how you perceive they view you. Our sense of self is reflected in and by others.

> After preparation ... Close your eyes and spend a little while with your breath. Don't change how you breathe (unless you wish to deepen it a little), but simply relax, letting the air easily flow in and out of your body ...
>
> Consider your relationships, not only the relationships with those closest to you, but also wider circles of friends, people at work, and so on ...
>
> Ask yourself: What is happening for me generally in these relationships? What is the nature of these relationships at the moment? ... What part do I play in these relationships? ...
>
> Ask yourself: How do I relate? ...

Begin to consider if there is any pattern to the way you relate with others, patterns of what you have been doing in relationships in your life. Can you sense any resemblance between current relationships and former ones? Or major differences? ...

Narrow your attention down to one or two of the most important relationships in your life. How do you see these people? How do they see you? ...

Ask yourself: How do I relate? ...

Do you recognise how you relate now in terms of life patterns set up earlier in life? ... [write]

How was your primary scenario? ...

How much are you still relating to and from that place? ... [write]

To be holistically healed you need to include the difficult relationships as well as the easy ones. When you are faced with difficult memories or experiences, do not rush for premature and therefore superficial healing in these relationships. Accept any difficulties that might arise as part of your experience, which can then inform your subsequent choices.

¶ BREAK

Love and connection

Psychosynthesis is not only involved with the individual, but also with groupings of people of all kinds. This encompasses our relationship with our parents, our children, our lovers and partners, our friends and colleagues and, on a wider level, all the groups to which we belong, including the whole of life. Psychosynthesis, understood as a natural process, encompasses all life, and one of its main aims is to create "right relations" between all beings.

Sometimes in our lives it is better to keep ourselves to ourselves and not share our energies. We do well to respect our inner wisdom when such times occur in our lives, and not to think or feel guilty if we choose to be separate or alone. At other times we feel more like exploring who we are and what we do as it relates to other people (and other beings).

Psychosynthesis offers a wealth of techniques and principles that can help us to facilitate this inner process. The very best way to explore our interpersonal expression, however, is quite simply through expressing ourselves. A good part of interpersonal relating is always trial and error, and it is through taking risks and exploring this arena that we can truly learn, grow and play a more active part in our "family".

> Reflect: Are there risks that you are not taking in your closest and most important relationships? ... [write]

Sometimes we do not express ourselves at all as we would wish. We start to express ourselves, then, depending upon the reaction we receive, we may stop altogether, suppress elements of our expression or totally change direction. This applies not only to individual situations but to how we interact overall with other people. Some people are "stopped altogether" most of the time and find it really hard to express themselves. Most of us suppress many different aspects of our inner world but do not express the totality of who we are with other people.

The first principle of interpersonal psychosynthesis is that the most important step to success is to accept ourselves for what we are. Once we accept ourselves without judgement or censorship, we can simply express who we are without holding back. Then we open up the possibility of change both individually and interpersonally. This does not mean we cannot or should not have secrets and, indeed, to respect the power of silence. Sometimes we share aspects of our growth and development too soon and thus dissipate some of the energy. Sometimes our "need" to relate makes us share things more from a level of deficiency rather than inclusion. Our secret inner world needs to be cherished and fostered, and kept secret. Then, when we are choosing to be intimate, we can allow others to share in some of this world, the power and awareness of which can be one of our major strengths.

A second major principle of interpersonal psychosynthesis is not to label people or "put them in boxes". If we want someone to stop seeing us in a certain way, we have to stop seeing them in that way. We can easily slip into seeing people in "boxes" instead of accepting the other person as they are. We then start relating to the box instead of the person. Then we don't have to be really present or take any real risks in opening ourselves up, for once we put someone else in a box, we put ourselves in a box too. Boxes are not noted for having great interpersonal relationships with one another! Fortunately, however, the opposite is also true: if we accept someone for what they are and do not label or box them, then we give them the space to treat us similarly well.

When we acknowledge another person and honour their uniqueness and individuality, we set the scene for true love to emerge. We also open up the possibility of change, which is often why we find it so scary to do this. If things change, we imagine we might lose out in some way so we cling to what is as if our lives depended upon it. Of course, in a sense, this is true, for when change occurs our lives do change. If we take the risk of letting others truly be themselves, though, then the likelihood is the change will be life-enhancing and positive. This is not always so easy, of course, but at least through trying we can move ourselves forward in a positive direction.

This leads us towards another major principle of interpersonal psychosynthesis, which is the understanding that to be loved, the only thing we have to give up is the experience of not being loved.

> After preparation ... Reflect: How are you with the experience of not being loved? ... Could you give this experience up easily? ... What are the obstacles to this? ... How can you honour these obstacles? ... [write]

---- ¶ BREAK ----

Projection and perception

We have a tendency to project onto other people, or the world in general, all the ideas and images, fantasies, feelings and thoughts that we have about other people and the world. This projection can take place consciously or unconsciously. In this way, we create our own reality, different, by the nature of this projection, from everyone else's reality. However, if we take a basic truth of interpersonal relationships, that it only takes one person to change the relationship, then if we start re-owning our projections, we create change. Then we may appreciate the differences between ourselves and other people, be willing to hear the good things people say about us as well as the bad, and give people good feedback when they do things that clearly honour us for who we are.

Basically, we have to accept another person for who they are, even if we cannot accept some aspects of their behaviour. There is a major difference between who someone is and what they do. Once we start relating to who they are then we are relating to them at a level of soul rather than just the personality. At this level all conflicts and disharmonies are full of potential growth. If we would like aspects of our relationship to be different then we cannot really blame anyone else but ourselves.

Of course, our personal reality is not just projection, there are many other components too, and what we have primarily to work with in any relationship is our perceptual reality. We create and live by our own beliefs and actions. If we can learn to stop projecting our feelings and start accepting them as ours, then we have taken a major step to improving our relationships and can start seeing the other people involved for who they really are. Then we move towards more of an "I–Thou" relationship where we can express ourselves clearly and allow the fuller expression of the other person or people involved.

> Reflect: Are there relational situations where you can see your interaction with one or more other people involves projection? ... [write]

--- ¶ BREAK ---

Mother activity

> Get an image of your mother (or the person who you knew in that role when very small) ... how does she look? How is she looking at you? What do you experience when she looks at you? ...
>
> Build the image more strongly, with more detail, allow it to become stronger ... How do you feel now before your mother? ... What do you want or need to say to her? ... What does she want or need to say to you? ... Enter into a dialogue with your mother, allowing yourself to experience all the different feelings and sensations that might emerge ... Continue the dialogue for as long as feels right to you ...
>
> It will soon be time to end this dialogue ... Is there anything you have been holding back from saying? ... Find an appropriate way now to end this dialogue ... [write]

Our relationship with mother is primary and forms both the basis of and pattern for all future relating. It is of course important to distinguish between the real mother out there (who might be absent, dead, even unknown) and the internalised inner mother of whom we speak here. The relationship to this "inner mother" is our connection with the mother archetype. There are different ways of responding to the mother archetype, as different as our inner experiences of her may be. For instance:

- The archetype becomes overdeveloped, leading to an overly strong maternal instinct, living through others, always giving, even when inappropriate.
- The erotic aspect of the relationship becomes overdeveloped, leading to obsessive behaviour around love, romance and sex, and a tendency to be always looking outside to find oneself.
- An identification where not being able to live up to her apparent standards leads to paralysis of emotional and mental functions, giving up, an inability to try things out.
- Resistance to mother, unconsciously acting out an attitude where we will do anything not to be like her.

We recognise such patterns through how we relate to those who trigger such a response, for example, our partners, but in particular how we mother ourselves and our inner child.

---------- ¶ BREAK ----------

A living extension

In its earliest months a new-born child is a living extension of its mother (or whomever or whatever plays the mother role for the baby). The mother and child live in a constant physical and energetic interchange. For the little one the first six months or so is lived in a world where there is no distinction between what is inside and what is outside, they are one and the same. This baby also lives in the illusion that it has created its world. A mother meanwhile (at least ideally) feels empathy, doesn't expect anything in return for her constant attention, and is basically dedicated to the survival and well-being of the baby. Many mothers report this unconditional love phase of the early relationship. Of course, this feeling, coming from the depths of her procreative archetype, will trigger the woman's own issues about oneness and separateness, so this period can bring great difficulties for her personally and within the relationship.

Then, around six months or so, this changes. The baby experiences a failure on the part of the mother, who is starting to noticeably withdraw and assert her separateness. She no longer attends to the baby's every need so the baby experiences the feeling of abandonment. This is inevitable and part of our human development. How present or absent the mother is, and how well she copes with this phase (both within herself and within the relationship) has a profound effect on the child's development. Our basic connection with the archetypes of oneness and separateness is programmed. One result of this is we internalise the image of mother, and split her into two parts, the good mother and the bad mother. Whatever our gender, the relationship with the feminine archetype is set.

As we go through further stages of development, what happens at this time will profoundly affect how the developing child (and adult) will deal with further transitional stages. By the time the infant has reached 18 months (or thereabouts) they will have learned the power of being able to say yes or no to things, the first steps in asserting independence. At this stage of development, how the yes and no responses are either inhibited or encouraged again affects the relationship to the mother archetype. It is established that good mother continues to nurture us while bad mother has abandoned us. Of course, different cultural attitudes and methods of bringing up infants, as well as gender differences also affect this. For instance, in a traditional Western culture, boys are more likely to be praised than girls for having an independent attitude.

The American psychologist Stan Grof created a model used by some psychosynthesis practitioners called the BPM Model. BPM stands for Basic Perinatal Matrices, so we are definitely better off sticking to BPM. There are four stages, BPM1 to BPM4. BPM1 is the stage of totally undifferentiated unity. The foetus is undisturbed within the womb. The beginning of separation signals BPM2. The foetus feels a movement, a pushing sensation. It feels trapped, limited, as if there is no way out. At some point the energy changes and the baby now responds by moving forward, towards the light at the end of the tunnel as it were. According to this model, the basic patterns within us for responsibility, assertion and autonomy are fixed at this stage. This is the stage called BPM3. BPM4 is that of the differentiated new-born and, in a sense, the individual throughout the rest of life, moving towards individuation and, eventually, a reunion. How this life is lived is dependent upon what was experienced during the earlier BPM stages and how these experiences are dealt with during the subsequent stages of development.

The following exercise, while not directly about birth, involves connecting with some of the energies of that time, and your subsequent experiences and responses to this.

> Your starting procedure should include some physical exercises to loosen and warm up your body. When you are ready, stand in a comfortable and relaxed position with as much space as possible around yourself.
> Imagine there is a wall surrounding you. Explore its surface (do this physically, starting with your hands) ... What is the wall made of—glass, stone, what? ...
> Feel the wall with your back ... feel it with your hips ... and feel it with any other parts of your body that seems right to you ... Is your wall really firm, or is it yielding? ... Does it feel alive or dead? ... What is the temperature of your wall? ...
> For you, having this wall around you, does it make you feel secure and comfortable, or does it make you feel restricted or trapped? ...
> Press against the wall, gently or with force, quickly or in a sustained manner, in whatever way feels right to you ... Is it resistant or flexible? Exaggerate how it feels with you pushing it ...
> Be sensitive to how you feel about the size, shape and resistance of your wall, its height and thickness ... stay in relationship with how you feel about your wall ...
> Now let the feeling of the wall remind you of some space you have been in before ... let the images, thoughts and feelings associated with this space emerge; do not judge or censor them, but only go as far with these feelings and images as feels appropriate to you at this moment ...
> Respond accordingly to these memories, letting your body move ...
> Come back to yourself, walk around a little, thoroughly shake off any unwanted energies and, only when you are ready, continue with the remainder of this activity ...
> Write about how you responded to the wall. Consider:
>
> - did you learn these responses as a child?
> - do these learned responses work?
> - did you get what you needed?

- what did you do about that?
- were you allowed to do this when you were a child?
- how did those around you respond when you acted like this?
- what else did you do? ... [write]

Our ego develops as a container for all our energies, to protect and support us through our lives. We should not denigrate our relationship with ego. Ego is not a good master but is an excellent friend. When we become totally identified with ego (a stage we all go through, and which people do not necessarily pass beyond) we live by our learned and adapted behaviour patterns based on a split between "me" and "other" predicated around fear and escape mechanisms. The useful container has become a limiting prison. We have built an ego to protect us, and now our unfulfilled needs control us. This is sometimes called the adapted personality. It is important part of our development for us to have a good, strong ego because it acts as a container for our growth and a vehicle for the experience and expression of our spiritual energies. The issue we have to be aware about is whether we have "got ego" or if ego has "got us".

¶ BREAK

From birth to adolescence

As we have been exploring, the process of birth involves a separation (from the womb) and a bonding (with mother). Most people continue to unconsciously and compulsively repeat patterns set up at this crucial time in an attempt to both meet their basic needs and to manifest the Self. These primal events will have affected your subsequent life, particularly in repeating cycles of behaviour. The underlying theme is the experience of oneness and separateness. These issues are key themes in psychosynthesis theory because they describe two opposite experiences that co-exist at the same time. We can recognise that we are both separate and at-one at the same time, our primary experience depending upon which pole we focus our attention. Looking at the processes of birth, bonding, oneness with and separation from mother, you can explore how you, as an individual, learned to be in the world, and negotiated your eventual separation from your mother, a process that happened in cycles and stages.

Our psychological birth or separation from mother is a time of primary importance, and part of a process that occupies much of our early infancy (from birth to three years old, sometimes called "the oral phase"). Including the experience of optimal failure by the mother (unconsciously creating "difference"), all this interaction sets the stage for the development of your personality. During our subsequent life, the pattern of experience set up at this time is then mostly experienced through the polarities of trust and mistrust.

When we can recognise two opposite experiences that co-exist within us, an opportunity opens for us to move to a third position from where we can observe the polarities and choose how the needs of both may be satisfied.

> After preparation ... Reflect on the following questions:
>
> Are you feeling at one with yourself today, or do you in any way feel separated from yourself? Tune into how you are feeling inside yourself right now ...
>
> Focus on your family ... to what extent do you feel one with your family, and to what extent do you feel separate from them? ...
>
> Now look at your relationships, both within your family and in your life generally ... Who are the people you feel at one with? ... who do you feel separate from? ...
>
> Now reflect on your relationship with your mother when you were a small child ...
>
> Did you feel at one with her or separate from her? In what ways did you and she merge? How was it for you as a small child to separate from your mother? ...
>
> Which do you fear more: Merging or separating? ...
>
> In your life do you avoid either of these experiences: To merge, to belong, to be involved in situations with people or to be on your own, self-sufficient, separate from others? ...
>
> Are both the need to merge and the need to be separate present in your personality? ... [write]

¶ BREAK

Childhood development

So much happens in an individual's development through childhood, and we are only dealing here with some of the issues that are most relevant to our current investigation. From birth until about two years of age is a time, primarily, for connecting to the basic archetypes of existence. These include the experience of birth itself, the meaning and purpose of incarnation, "having a new start", and so on. The actual experiences undergone during this period around these archetypal energies, which will persist through life. For instance, how you view and relate to your purpose for being here, and how you deal with new beginnings in your life will be set up at this time.

Most early relating, certainly that of greatest significance, is with your parents. On this primary level you learn how much you can trust (or mistrust) the world around you. If our relationship with our parental figures was clearly formed, then we know it is okay to be ourselves (to love ourselves) and it is okay to change (to empower ourselves). If these relationships were not so clearly defined, and in most of us this is exactly the case, then we exhibit corresponding distortions. We need to ask ourselves exactly what did our parents teach us about love and power? And we need to remember that were not victims to some "horrible ogres" whose conscious or unconscious aim was to cause us pain in later life. It is always true that, whatever we do, it is the best we can do at that time. This is equally true of other people, including our parents or guardians.

Realising this brings acceptance, and true acceptance, as we have already learned, brings clarity to our ability to be ourselves, and our ability to be both loving and wilful. Just as we can bless any apparent obstacle to our growth and development, so we can bless our parents for doing the best they could. Forgiveness removes any lack of wholeness. Forgiveness brings love both to the person forgiven and to the forgiver. We can never have enough forgiveness.

> After preparation, reflect: What is it like for you when you trust yourself, others, and your environment? ...
> When you are trusting with your body, what do you sense and feel? ...
> Now turns your attention to mistrust: What is it like for you when you mistrust yourself, others, and your environment? ...

How do you experience mistrust in body; what do you sense and feel? ...

How do you relate to people differently when you are in these different modes? ... [write]

Now reflect: What is your ongoing relationship like with trust and mistrust? ...

Which do you identify with more, being trusting or mistrusting? ...

How do you experience being trusting and mistrusting? ...

What are the behaviours you exhibit with trusting and mistrusting? ...

Describe in some detail two of your subpersonalities, one who is a trusting type, and one who is a mistrusting type (e.g. the merger and the avoider) ... [write]

Consider the importance of having both these subpersonalities.

Reflect: Is there more energy in the one with which you usually identify less? ...

Are both polarities important in your life? Where do you choose to place yourself now? ... [write]

¶ BREAK

The expression of love

We can love ourselves or other people either from our sense of self, our centre, or in a more partial way, perhaps from a needy subpersonality. There is nothing wrong with loving someone in a partial way so long as we do not become identified with it in a way that does them or us a disservice. When we love from our centre, however, we can be more objective, loving without attachment, caring but not overwhelming, strong but not manipulative.

To love from a subpersonality usually involves various aspects of need—I love you because you give me something or other. It depends upon the response—I won't love you any more unless you continue giving me whatever it is. To love from the self is to be proactive rather than reactive, to love someone for who and what they are rather than what they do. To be able to say I still love you despite what you are doing. Love from a subpersonality is usually shallower and more whimsical whereas love from the self is deeper and more lasting. Love from the centre is whole rather than partial, complete rather than fragmented. It is a synthesis of love and will, thinking, feeling and sensing. In this way it is complete and gives a sense of freedom rather than bondage.

We may try to understand love through analysing it in this way, but it is still love, however. Love quite simply just is. If it comes through a subpersonality, it may be less whole, more needy, more reactive, but it is still love, and we have the power within us to change it, to transform it into a more centred love. If we consciously work on meeting the needs of a subpersonality, it can change and become more self-sufficient. When this happens, the love this subpersonality expresses can also become more self-sufficient. Parts of us that feel little or no love can have their "love element" expanded while parts of us that have lots of love but express it in a distorted way can have their "love element" refined. It is always worth stressing again that this a basic principle for all psychosynthesis work, that we can elevate or expand energies we have too little of and refine or purify those energies of which we have too much.

When we realise and express love, we find its qualities abound. True love, of ourselves or others, gives us the energy for creative acts, it gives us insights and confidence, it strengthens and nourishes us, and, perhaps most importantly, it allows us to discover more about our true, inner selves. Often it is more difficult to realise and express self-love than it is to express love to others. Yet how much richer and more meaningful our lives become if we allow ourselves some self-love. This does not mean narcissistically becoming enamoured of our bodies, our emotions, feelings, thoughts or even our deepest soul connections. What it does mean is to accept ourselves for what we are, in totality, and realise we are what we are, nothing more or nothing less. When we accept ourselves, we realise the greatest love within and are more able to express it.

Love in itself is often not enough, however, and it has to be coupled with understanding otherwise it can blindly cause problems where it aims to release, can maim and spoil where it intends to free and encourage, can become sentimentality instead of simply being itself. Love to be truly helpful has to be applied with wisdom and understanding.

If we see only our own viewpoint and do not truly see the position of others, then we are obscuring the free flow of love. If we assert ourselves at the expense of others, in an artificial, excessive or inappropriate way, then we block love. If we have prejudices and preconceived ideas about how love should be expressed then we block love that way too. But if we let love flow through us as channels for its greater energy, and if we work on making ourselves more conscious and more efficient channels for this energy, then love is our sustenance and salvation.

There is no such thing as an "ideal relationship", but we can all consciously choose to create a reality in which we move towards rather than away from such a goal. In an ideal relationship we relate primarily in a holistic way. This means we include all parts of our personality, including the darker parts. We see the other person or people involved as equally whole and love them unconditionally. We own our shadows, and do not project it onto others. We love without need or deficiency, and are willing to surrender to how the relationship evolves. We can move towards this ideal in all our relationships, but for it to become the primary focus we have to work at it, not because we think we should but because we really want to.

---¶ BREAK---

A true meeting

The following exercise is powerful and can be deeply moving. You can adapt this exercise to try face to face with an actual person if you like, but familiarise yourself with it in imagination first.

> After preparation ... Consider someone with whom you have (or would very much like) a deep, meaningful and positive relationship ...
>
> Imagine sitting opposite this person, letting yourself build up a big picture just as if they are there ... use senses to make them as real as possible. As well as how they appear visibly to you, how does this person smell? taste? What do they sound like? How would you feel to be touching them? ...
>
> As you sit opposite this person acknowledge all the protections that are available to you, and affirm that you have a choice to be as much or as little protected as you like ...

Notice what your responses and reactions are to sitting before this person, imagining you maintain a steady eye contact throughout. Include your feelings of embarrassment, fear, sexuality, vulnerability, excitement, whatever …

Ask yourself: What is it of myself I am able to show? … What of myself am I not yet ready to show? … [write]

Imagine the person again. Imagine what it would be like to see this person now from your heart. Affirm a willingness to open a little more to this person … Keep breathing into your heart area, and as you do this remember you still have a choice …

As you look at this person before you, be aware of their many layers: appearance, physical shape, hands, dress, behaviour, what they look like, how you've seen them … Imagine all these layers painted on glass …

Keep looking and begin to see through all these layers on the glass until you get deeper to the essence of this person. See layers drop away. Feel your own layers similarly drop away …

As you get deeper and deeper you experience the essence of this person …

As you connect to the essence of this person be aware of your own essence …

Be aware you always have a choice about how much you see and how much you show …

Stay with this for a while …

Now visualising the person again clearly, gently say goodbye to them. Be aware of how attached or not you are to holding on, and choose to let go for now …

Really come back to yourself. Be aware of being with yourself …

Do something to ground yourself …

Remember you may have seen this person's essence in this exercise, but that doesn't mean in the ordinary everyday world you can just drop your boundaries. Respond appropriately to what you have experienced in this exercise and the real person out there. Relationships are a mystery, an exciting mystery to be lived and not worked out intellectually.

--- ¶ BREAK ---

Choices to make

After preparation ... Connect to a sense of goodwill towards yourself. Based on your experiences in this lesson, are there any choices you need to make in relation to yourself and the relationships in your life? ...

If it is right for you, affirm your choices to yourself. Act appropriately.

–––––––––––––––––––– ¶ BREAK ––––––––––––––––––––

Before starting the next lesson

- Continue to reflect on your relationship with your subpersonalities, particularly as they interact with other people with whom you are in relationship. Don't make this judgemental, simply observe the responses and reactions of your subpersonalities to the behaviour of others' subpersonalities, and vice versa.
- Give yourself at least one hour during which time you cannot be interrupted. Spend this time considering your current relationships in light of what you've been exploring in this lesson.

LESSON 5

The child of wisdom: the inner child and family dynamics

This lesson focuses on building a stronger and more healing relationship with your inner child. Your inner child is the repository of your earliest memories, feelings and experiences, often associated with the trauma and stress of early development, as we have been exploring. While these early experiences may have caused wounds, we find they also hold wisdom and creativity. How your inner child learned to deal with the world wasn't pathological; it was their function to ensure you survived, and so they learned to behave in ways that attempted to ensure that survival. As adults, we carry round this inner child (or inner children) within us, affecting how we behave and interact now in our lives.

You are guided through exercises to connect with your family of origin, explore your early experiences, and engage in a dialogue with your inner child. By doing so, you can address past wounds, find meaning in your life, and align with your soul's guidance. Additionally, the lesson delves further into the phases of childhood development, emphasising the importance of these formative years and how they shape our adult selves. The text underscores that each of us has unique wounds, and that befriending and attending to your inner child can lead to greater happiness and effectiveness as an adult.

Our exploration of the journey of life now reaches adulthood, and we look at how we move back and forth in our experience of life as our development moves between progress and regression. We also explore the difference between how we experience the crises that, as it were, repeat or hark back to our childhood and those of a more immediate existential origin.

Finally, we also touch on sexuality and identity, emphasising the importance of integrating sexuality into one's life in a balanced and conscious manner. You are asked to revisit and question your beliefs, as they are often formed in childhood and can influence your perception of the world. Through revisiting and revising these constructs, you can find greater clarity and understanding, aligning with your true self and the wisdom of your soul.

Review

Did you give yourself at least one uninterrupted hour considering your current relationships? If not, reflect (and write) on your reasons for this. For instance, your reflection might consider subpersonalities that support your progress in self-development and those who find it fearful. Which subpersonalities encouraged you to take time for yourself and which, for instance, kept you too busy doing other things to do so? Remember, this is not about making judgements on yourself, or you being judged in any way, but to help you to uncover more of the workings of your psyche.

--- ¶ BREAK ---

Back in the family

Imagine yourself back in your family of origin (which most usually involves a mother, usually a father, other close family members, even close family friends, and so on, but may, of course, not necessarily involve any of these. The people with whom you grew up are your family of origin) … imagine yourself in relationship with these different characters, for now not focusing on the relationship with particular people, but the sense of being in relationship with your whole family …

THE CHILD OF WISDOM

Allow an image to emerge in your mind that represents this relationship; don't censor or judge, but trust the image that first comes to you ... allow time for it to develop (if appropriate), and then bring your consciousness clearly back to your body ...

Draw this image or make a record of it as appropriate. The drawing doesn't so much have to be an exact replica of whatever image you received, more a representation of your relationship to that image ... [write]

After finishing the drawing, write a little on the attitude towards you of the different members of your extended family. How do their attitudes towards you affect you now? ... [write]

———————————— ¶ BREAK ————————————

Relating to the child within

The child within exists and develops in relationship to its family of origin.

After preparation ... Imagine yourself back in your family situation, the family you grew up in, and the environment of your early years ... allow yourself to recall these times as vividly as you are able ...

Notice reactions in your body to doing this ...

Don't try to change any feelings or emotions that come up, but include them ... How do you feel as you imagine yourself back in this family, as a child? ...

Ask yourself: In those days, did anyone take delight in me, and take pleasure in my presence? If so, whom? If not, what was that like for you? ...

What messages did you receive about how you should and should not be? ... Was it okay to be sad, or angry, or to show other emotions? Was it okay to have needs? ...

Imagine yourself standing outside and in front of the first or earliest remembered place you lived ("the house of the past"). Notice your sensations and feelings ...

Imagine the door opens and you see in the doorway a little child. Notice your first impulse but do not act upon it ... Spend some time allowing the child to become more clearly visible to you ...

How do you feel meeting this child? ... If it feels okay, allow this child to take you to a safe place where the two of you can be alone ... Feel what it is like for you to be in the presence of this child. Take some time to talk to one another about your relationship with one another and whatever else come up ... Is there anything the child wishes to say that has been unspoken? ...

Is there anything you want to say to the child that you have never said? ...

How do you feel now about this child? ... What, if anything, do you recognise this child needs? ... Is there anything you can do about that right now, or soon? ...

Pay attention to what the child really needs ...

Acknowledge to this child that you can and will return and meet again if you both wish ... Find some way for now to say goodbye for now to the child ... [write]

Ground yourself in some way after this exercise, including in this the needs of your child.

Make sure you take a good long break, staying with your feelings for a while after this experience.

¶ BREAK

Growing the child within

The phases of life's journey most relevant to the development of the inner child are the first four—those we have called baby, toddler, child and adolescent (see diagram 4 on p. 29). They could be described as the four phases of childhood. (If you are familiar with other models of child development you will have already seen how this model simplifies other theories.) To summarise:

- The baby stage (roughly 0 to 6 months) is primarily concerned with issues of trust (and mistrust). The baby is involved in symbiotic bonding and does not consider the outside world and inside world as separate. The tasks of this stage are survival and growth.
- The toddler stage (roughly 6 months to 2 years) is primarily concerned with issues of autonomy (and shame and doubt). The toddler is involved in oppositional bonding, being now aware that there is a

self and an outside world to interact with. The tasks of this stage are exploration and separation.
- The child stage (roughly 2 years to puberty) is primarily concerned with issues of self-worth (and self-deprecation). The child is involved in trusting the world and building ego strength through interdependence and cooperation issues. The tasks of this stage are learning and relating.
- The adolescent/teenager (from puberty to "leaving home") is primarily concerned with issues of ego identity (and role confusion). The teenager is involved in regeneration, finding their own sense of self in an unsupportive world and creating an independence from family. The tasks at this stage is learning to trust one's senses and being true to one's own inner sense of self.

Of course, in an ideal world this development would all happen apace and the young adult leaving home would be trusting, autonomous, have a sense of self-worth and be able to be self-reliant and interdependent as appropriate. To a greater or lesser degree, but with certainty, no one develops without events happening that wound the inner child and create breaks in this development. From a transpersonal perspective, we can say these wounds are the soul's way of creating the right situation for the learning it needs in this life. This is, however, in no way to lessen the pain and suffering that happens for us all, or to suggest we choose to be mistreated or abused. We can learn to honour our wounding without trying to pretend everything is all right. The aim in psychosynthesis is not to pretend wounds do not exist but to find ways to include the wounding so we can be more whole.

What happens to break the developmental pattern? Children are naturally filled with wonder, are optimistic, straightforward, dependent, emotionally alive, resilient, playful, unique and loving. The shadow-side of these traits are many: for example, wonderment can be inhibited and turned to fear by parents who are already closed-down; optimism can be broken by the abuse of trust; straightforwardness can be bent by too high or low expectations from the parents; vulnerability and dependence can be misused by the behaviour of a needy adult; emotional openness can be shamed and turned to sorrow and pain; resilience can be smashed on the arid shores of discouragement; playfulness can be corrupted and judged as wrong; the dignity of uniqueness can be subsumed by the absence of proper mirroring; love can be hurt by deprivations that leave only a faint echo of its power.

We are all wounded, in our own unique ways, during our childhood. We lose, in one or many ways, our sense of I-ness, our sense of self. We are wounded by neurotic and damaged parents and other adults, sometimes consciously but most often unconsciously. Sexual, physical and emotional abuse are the three main areas of abuse of the child. This can come from parents, other adults, siblings, at school, at other meetings, and not only from individuals but from the culture as a whole. Many of us have been shamed and led to believe we are not okay for being poor, or the wrong shape or size, wrong gender and so on. The ego is diminished, as it were, and we become lesser than our potential. You feel there is something wrong with you, and you cannot do anything about it.

Our early and unmet needs control us now. How important then to befriend your inner child and attend to her or his wants and needs. Then some little of the Quality at the core of being can be released, not only for the well-being of the child but for the whole organism. An adult with a befriended inner child is a much happier and more effective human than one who doesn't acknowledge or attend to the needs of this child. As with an outer child, the adult must set appropriate boundaries to protect the child, to honour them for their uniqueness; to be encouraging and engender a sense of trust; to be a good parent. Then the child can feel safe and supported to share their wisdom and understanding.

¶ BREAK

Revealing appearances

After preparation ... Reflect: How do you reveal yourself with your choice of clothes and body appearance (including any make-up, etc.)? ... What style do you adopt? ... What are you wearing? ... How did you choose this style and these clothes? ... Was your inner child involved in the choice? ... What other parts of yourself were involved? ...

Is the clothing you are wearing right now typical? How? Why (or why not)? ... What colours are you wearing? ... What meaning have these colours for you? ... What is your hair style? ... Are you wearing perfume? ... Ornaments, brooches, necklaces, watches, etc.? What about your underwear and clothing not generally intended to be seen by others—how have you chosen this? ...

Considering your appearance and clothing, what are you choosing to reveal about yourself? ... and to conceal? ... [write]

Another aspect of ourselves that reveals and conceals us is our name. Say your name out loud a few times ... What do you hear? ... How do you feel saying your name? ... Is this the name by which you were usually called in childhood? ... Say that name out loud a few times (if it is the same name, repeat it a few more times now) ... How does your inner child feel to have their name spoken out ... [write]

Reflect: How did you get your name? ... Have you changed your name in any way? ... How and under what circumstances did this happen? ... What effect have other people had on what you call yourself? ... What about your surname—what is its origins, and does it have a meaning? ... Do you connect with this name? ...

Close your eyes and inwardly say the name of your inner child in the sweetest, most loving tone you can ... Keep this up until your emotions tell you to stop ... how does your inner child feel now? ... [write]

---¶ BREAK---

Standing on the corner

The inner child has two aspects that we call the child of the past and the child of the future.

After preparation ... In your imagination, with your eyes closed, become your inner child ... allow yourself to take on the feelings, sensations and thoughts of this child as much as feels okay to you right now ...

Imagine, as this child, you are standing on a street corner. Spend some time getting a sense of this, visualising yourself at this corner ...

Looking back, you can see the house of the past and looking forward you can see the house of the future ...

What does the house of the past look like? ... How does it make you feel, looking at this house? ...

What does the house of the future look like? ... How does it make you feel, looking at this house? ...

Acknowledge in an appropriate way where you have come from, turn towards the house of the future and take a step in that direction ... [write]

Listen to the needs of your inner child ... and take them with you as you step forward ... Bring your awareness fully back into your body and, before doing anything else, find something to do which grounds you very firmly in your body and everyday world.

─────────────── ¶ BREAK ───────────────

Renewal, change and return

While we live with our inner child through our whole life, we also develop and grow older. We now turn to adult life, and in particular existential and mid-life crises. We all experience these crises throughout our life, repeating the cyclical patterns we have been exploring. It is not only the young child who "lives" within us, we also carry within the events, positive and negative in character, that have affected us in all the subsequent stages of our growth. So-called mid-life crisis, for instance, can occur any time from thirty to sixty years old, and may indeed be an ongoing theme throughout all these years. Certainly, we all have "crises of existence", times when we find life too difficult, meaningless, empty, or we lose track of ourselves and any sense of purpose.

Unlike any of our experiences that are determined by the past, for instance our fear of abandonment because mother left us in the pram, and so on, existential crises are more about the present and future (the middle and higher unconscious in the egg diagram—see p. 33). What we embark upon now in this course as well as in life is markedly different from what we have explored so far. We are focusing more with what comes after ego, the emergence and "growth" of soul. Of course, the past is still very relevant, because what we experience in our existential crises mirrors energies from the past, unresolved "stuff" brought up once again for us to face and—hopefully—deal with.

Existential crises can be seen as happening in three stages. Firstly, there is a separation from what has been in one's life before, the comfortable or at least familiar patterns of daily life. Finally, after the crisis, there is a return to the old life, but renewed by the experience. The stage in the middle—sometimes called "liminality"—is what concerns us most. The "limen" is the doorway, so to be in liminality means simply to be in a doorway, neither where you were before, nor where you are going afterwards.

> After preparation ... Reflect: What makes you feel comfortable in your life? ... What are you identified with, attached to in your life? ... What makes you feel secure? What makes you safe? What are you bonded to or attached to in order to get that security? ...
> Is this enough? ... [write]
> What in this security frustrates, constricts, holds you in bondage? ... What is missing when you are at home? ... What is missing when away from home? ... What's the question you need to ask yourself about your life right now? ... [write]
> From a developmental viewpoint, you are an adult now. You are living your life, you've left home and so on, or you have "made your arrangements" to live your life, then an existential, or a mid-life crisis arrives, and deep, life-challenging questions come up: Why am I here? What value am I? What is life for? And so on ... [write]
> Reflect for a moment: Is there life beyond ego?

Each transition and crisis we experience is an opportunity to re-centre at the core, our "self" or "I", or to remain in continuing reaction to the past, controlled by ego. This is not to suggest anything negative about ego; rather the issue is whether ego acts as an unkind master or as a trusted friend. The psychosynthesis egg diagram shows us how we need both, the ego forming a "bridge" between the self and the earth and body (the periphery of the egg). Ego depends upon the (past) contents of consciousness; the self is unique and exists without content.

As we go through our adult developmental stages, we walk a path between ego and self, becoming fixed in some places, avoiding others, having peak experiences that "take us up to the self", sometimes being "drawn down into the depths". Both experiences are of equal importance, and the true unattached self may be found in either.

An important aspect of the journey of life is to have companionship, whether this is close loved ones or fellow travellers we hardly know. It is important to be able to recognise others on the journey and let them recognise you too. In other words, our journey is enhanced through compassion and heart energy. While our wounding is unique to us, it mirrors or corresponds to the wounding of the world and the universe. We often read today about the wounded planet. If our individual wounds bring us closer to soul energy, then perhaps our collective and planetary wounds can do the same.

Some psychosynthesis theorists suggest we come into incarnation so we can learn lessons useful to our soul's journey. This is the purpose for our being here. Within this overriding life purpose, we take many smaller steps towards this unfoldment, and each small step is vitally important. We cannot take each step with an awareness of the bigger picture, but we can hold this as an underlying intent. Our birth memories, and memories and experiences from the early stages of our life, act as models for the rest of our lives, enabling a shift from a victim position towards a holistic vision where each cycle contains the pattern of the whole.

Two more of the many polarities we consider in psychosynthesis are differentiation and integration. Life is a search for and discovery of self, experienced through a constant polarity between moving forwards into life and/or backwards towards the womb. At all stages we become identified or attached to our experiences, and it is necessary for us to engage with these experiences and learn to differentiate. We forget; so, conversely, we are offered the opportunity to remember. To re-member is to put ourselves back together through an act of disidentification that enables us to move towards union with consciousness and choice.

Moments of crisis force an awakening in the journey, or sometimes we have moments of spontaneous awakening. We realise at these times of awakening that we are on a journey back home and may learn to hold an awareness of self as both separate and together at the same time. The journey of psychosynthesis is an adventure, a quest for determination and courage as old as humanity itself. The challenge of knowing oneself is the challenge of life, and psychosynthesis is a potent asset for getting to know oneself.

¶ BREAK

Sexuality and identity

Sex has three aspects: the physical and energetic aspect (corresponding to how we relate to the body and the external world as objects); the intra-personal aspect (corresponding to our relationship with ourselves, and our body as a somatic experience); and the inter-personal aspect (corresponding to our relationship with others). These aspects invariably (and inevitably) go together and the relationship between our inner and outer worlds is inexorably linked. For instance, an important aspect of our early development involves the bonding and mirroring that takes place helping us to form a sense of self. Issues arise through, for instance, desertion, lack of touch, isolation, or at the most extreme, physical abuse. In terms of our relationship to sexuality this may bring a fear of abandonment, behaviour controlled by a desperate need for closeness, or fear of intimacy.

How present we are able to be when we are in contact with another person is very dependent upon what has happened during our childhood development (well before adolescence). For instance, a child who has learned to restrict the normal expression of energy (to protect themselves in some way) splits off or creates their own separate world. This may then be repeated through being cut-off or going into observer role during sexual experiences. How we breathe directly relates to our emotional state and level of excitement. Splitting off often leads to inhibited breathing (possibly leading to many different psychosexual issues arising).

If containment and boundary issues around the expression of sexuality become disturbed, one common energetic result is that sexual arousal is equated with inevitable sexual activity. The experience of sexuality and the act of sex are linked. This can lead to acting out through inappropriate sexual behaviour. It cannot be emphasised too much that sexual arousal need not inevitably lead to sexual activity.

Sensuality involves not just the genitals and secondary sexual areas but the whole body. It is the experience of sexual energy without splitting off or acting out, without thinking and fantasy interrupting the energetic flow. It has to include all the pain, remorse, disappointment, longing, and other shadowy emotions and feelings to be truly whole. Many people try through sex to meet unfulfilled needs for intimacy, touch, tenderness and belonging, to feel better about themselves and how they relate to the world. Some people use sex to assert power and to act out in ways that are abusive both to themselves and others.

To understand the sexual component in any relationship, we need to explore the meaning and intention within the relationship, which can be positive or negative in actuality if not with intent. To isolate sexuality is not the most effective way to do this; we can better see sexuality as part of the whole picture. All our negative patterns, for example our resistance to the self, our identifications, our fears and so on, all are played out in sexual relating. But sex can also be viewed as spiritual, as a holy act of union between people. When one and one come together sex does not give us two, it gives us a newly formed, ecstatic one again. Our inner desire for Unity can be met and fulfilled through a positive attitude towards sex. A healthy open attitude can allow us to be ourselves in a new, exciting way, honouring primarily our relationship to ourselves and our own values. The most important issue is to bring awareness to play in your sexual life, then to apply all the principles you have learned for improving your own life to anyone else involved in your sexual sphere.

> After preparation ... Visualise a door with the word "sexuality" on it. Imagine opening this door and looking through to see what is on the other side. View what is there in detail. If you feel willing to do so, step into this other world and explore what is there. It is the realm of your own sexuality ...
>
> When you are ready, come back from this vision and distinctly and firmly close the door shut behind you. Return to your ordinary consciousness ...
>
> Consider what you saw in your vision of sexuality. Consider what your other senses told you about this place, and how you felt there ...
>
> Look for the qualities present behind the forms of what you saw. Look for aspects of union. Did you see emotional patterns reflected in your vision? How is your self-image reflected there? Did you identify with what you saw, and are you able to disidentify from it? ...
>
> Consider: What is the meaning you put on your sexuality? What attitudes and concepts do you hold about your sexuality? ... [write]

The psychosynthesis attitude to sexuality stresses that most sexual problems fall into one or other of two categories: not operating sexually (too little), and only operating sexually (too much). A worthwhile approach to transforming sexuality is simply putting it into perspective. Rather than sexuality "having us" we can learn to have it. We have sexuality so we can use it (not that sexuality has us so it can "use" us!). Of course, as always disidentification should not be used as a means of avoidance. To "have sexuality" you must be coming from a genuinely disidentified place or you cannot choose to let go and surrender to it when that is appropriate. To transform sexuality and our relationship with it, the areas we need to focus on are the belly and heart, and, in this sense, also the relationship between ego and self. We investigate these best through looking at sexuality as we experience it in the present, at least as much as is possible considering all the misinformation, conditioning, control, and worse, we live through these days.

It is always worth reminding oneself that sexual energy is life energy; we would not be here without it, and despite all the limitations we experience, sexuality is a positive force that brings not only pleasure and sometimes pain, but it is, at core, the very energy that brought us to life in the first place.

¶ BREAK

Developing meaning

As an adult you can create a deeper and more meaningful relationship with your inner child, while through this you are at the same time building a greater understanding between you and your soul. What your soul tells you through the child will be the truth, but the way you hear the message can be distorted, so take care in how you interpret anything you receive. It is important to discriminate, to look for non-verbal reinforcement, any changes in body position or breath patterns that suggest whether the dialogue is working effectively. Also watch for judgements creeping in—the soul is never judgemental towards the personality—firm yes, but angry, no.

Try to find ways to express in your daily life what the soul tells you so you can check its validity in the real world. Remember you are the soul and you have a personality, not vice versa. Don't worry if this doesn't work too well for you, it certainly does not mean you are without a soul.

It might be simply that the exercise is not right for you in some way, or it might be that, at this time in your personal evolution, your soul is choosing to work "undercover" and a dialogue would be inappropriate. Trust that your own process is unfolding as it is meant to, and you cannot go far wrong.

> Reflect back over this day and ask yourself: What am I doing here? What is the meaning in all the things I have done today? Try to perceive an underlying pattern behind all areas of action and focus through your day. Spend some time on this, reflecting on these emerging patterns and actions in life …
>
> Now abstract from this particular day and see the events you have been considering within a wider context. See your life as a whole … [write]

Everything you think is a belief, a mental construct. What time of day is it? What day of the week? Answers to all such questions involve a belief, a mental construct about the meaning of time and space, being here as opposed to there, being now as opposed to then. Being on this beautiful planet in this vast universe is also a construct; everything is a construct. Being in a galaxy, on a planet, in a house, in this room, all these ideas are constructs. The kind of person you believe you are—this is a construct, different from the simple perception of being. The world you live in, this is a construct, too. Remember that constructs are not "real" in any concrete sense and can be changed. Do you like the world you live in? Do you like the "game" you are playing?

Some constructs can seem more right than others. Look for this rightness, and hold these constructs; let others go, and constantly revise your position on what you "know" to be true, what you believe in and what you don't. If you are not flexible you are rigid, and rigid things break under stress. A Taoist sage once told a monk that a twisted tree they were passing was very wise. When asked to explain, he said that the trees that grow up perfectly straight and strong get cut down for use as firewood, for furniture, boats or whatever. This tree, by going with the flow of nature, bending this way with the winds and that way with the rains, had grown up twisted and gnarled, but had been left to its own devices, to grow as it chose, and had not been cut down or used. Its trust in the flow of nature had ensured it a long life.

You can find those moments when you connect with a sense of rightness. This is a form of intuition, of which there are basically three kinds:

- "I know but I don't know why"—a kind of common sense that comes through your thoughts, feelings or body. We often distrust these intuitions as being "fantasy" or imagination, which of course sometimes they are. On the other hand, though, we can learn to separate those we can trust from those that are fantasies through using our discriminative faculties. If you still yourself and look at your thoughts and feelings about a situation, sometimes it becomes easier to tell if this "knowing" is genuine intuition or something you have created in your imagination without a connection to a deeper level of knowledge.
- "I have a sense it is right"—this "sense" comes into the superconscious, and is to do with rightness and choice. For it to manifest, you have to look at the most holistic, largest vision you hold. Without a connection to this larger picture, it is too easy to have all kinds of "senses" about situations or people that are way off the mark. If you hold your connection to your deeper or innermost self, then you can trust that your intuitions are in line with "the highest good".
- "It came to me in a flash"—these intuitions include major insights, glimpses of an intuitive plan at the highest level, and can manifest directly or through great music, works of art or even in the most unexpected and strange ways, for example, when synchronistic events occur or strange connections are made between you and someone or something else. The nature of this kind of intuitive insight leaves little doubt about the veracity of its message, for a true "flash" enters your consciousness with enough light to make itself felt in an unambiguous way. If there is any ambiguity then you have to question where the intuition came from and whether it is truly guidance from the soul.

All your beliefs or "worldviews" you probably learned as a child, from parents, the church, school teachers and so on. You might not consciously believe them anymore, but unless you work on them, they are still there as unconscious constructs and will affect your life, and can at least potentially, and, in most cases, definitely hold you back from expressing who you truly are. And it is essential to remember there is no right answer to anything, just different points of view. It is important to watch for assumptions in this process. For example, fear is an assumption something will go wrong, or at least possibly go wrong. Can it?

Mistrust is an assumption that there is not an order and a plan in the universe. Isn't there? How do you know either way? Frustration is an assumption that there is an alternative way to do things. Yet if there is an alternative way of doing things, what is there to be frustrated about?

If a construct is a map then it is fine, it can help you find out where you are and connect you to where you wish to go. On the other hand, if it affects and colours the territory then it is no longer enhancing to you or your life. It is all as simple and as complicated as that!

> Reflect deeply about everything you know: people, places, anything that comes to mind. Allow your thoughts to run as free associations, without censoring anything and, as far as possible, without judging anything. Let this process continue for some time, then ask: Who is aware of all these thoughts? ... [write]

There is only one being, there is only one awareness. This unity is becoming increasingly manifest. Soul is increasingly manifesting through you. Come back into your life with this awareness and ground it.

¶ BREAK

Into the heart

> After preparation ... Be aware of how you are feeling now, as an adult, about yourself and your inner child at this time in your life development, at whatever stage you happen to be ... don't try and push anyway any feelings, however you experience them, but include them ...
>
> Imagine you can once again see your inner child in front of you. Notice how you feel ... In your imagination, open your arms wide and take this child into your heart ... Remain in silence with this child for as long as you both wish ...
>
> When you are ready: ... [write]
>
> To end this meditation, take yourself and your inner child to some place or to do something you will both enjoy doing together.
>
> After you return: [write] about this experience.

¶ BREAK

Before starting the next lesson

- Continue to stay in close touch with your inner child, particularly during interactions with other people. Don't make this judgemental, simply observe the responses and reactions of your inner child to the behaviour of others' subpersonalities, and vice versa.
- Give yourself at least one hour during which time you cannot be interrupted. Spend this time considering your current stage of life in light of what you've been exploring in this lesson.

LESSON 6

The art of self-identification: becoming the conductor of your life

This lesson discusses the concept of identification and its influence on our lives. It emphasises that we are identified with various aspects of ourselves, such as self-image, beliefs, feelings, and more. These identifications change over time, and our goal is to become less identified with those that no longer serve us. You are encouraged to recognise some of your major identifications, to work on disidentification from these and shift to identifying with your core self from where you can make your best choices. The aim is to have a balanced relationship with all aspects of your being.

The most important practice in psychosynthesis is introduced, the self-identification exercise, which guides you in disidentifying from the contents of your personality and towards identifying with the self. We start then to explore the developmental stages of life from a deeper, soul-centred perspective and how different functions come to the foreground at various ages.

Working on achieving a balanced relationship with all our functions is crucial for our holistic development at all stages of life, and such a balance can be effectively found and maintained effectively through self-identification with the "I", the "conductor" for the rest of the personality, the "orchestra".

Finally, a detailed description of how meditation is used in psychosynthesis is followed by an exploration of the inner guide, a source of wisdom that helps us navigate our growth and integration. This dialogue can offer guidance in various life situations, helping us make choices aligned with our deeper life purpose, and finding ways to express that purpose in life.

Review

Did you give yourself at least one uninterrupted hour considering your relationship with your inner child, particularly in relation to your interaction with other people? If not, reflect (and write) on your reasons for this. I think I've said it often enough by now, but do remember this review is not about judgement but insight into how your psyche operates.

Past identifications

Whatever we are identified with controls us. We are all identified with our self-image(s), view of the world, specific beliefs, attitudes, feelings, sensations and so on. These identifications change as we go through life. What is important at one time, for example a particular religious belief, a relationship, a way of being in the world, a feeling that we need to protect ourselves, may become less important at another time of life. This is because we have disidentified from this belief or feeling so we are no longer attached in the same way. For instance: I might still care for the person I was previously attached to, but I am no longer obsessively in love; I can't imagine how I was so completely involved in that religion; and so on.

So far, we have looked at some of the components of our psychic make-up: body, feelings, mind, subpersonalities and the inner child (or perhaps, more correctly, inner children). We have many faces we show to the world, and many we keep hidden. With any or all of these parts of ourselves, it is possible to become stuck with it. At times some parts of us might appear to take us over, as it were, and it was only later, depending upon how identified we were, that we notice how totally caught up we were in being a victim in that situation.

> After preparation ... Reflect on times in your past where you have been strongly identified with something (whether feelings, beliefs,

or attitudes). What was it like to be caught up in this way, and what changed to make you less identified? ... [write]

---- ¶ BREAK ----

Believe it or not

We all have beliefs about who we are (for instance: I am a good person, I am a rebel, I am no good, I am a teacher, I am stupid, I am... and so on) These beliefs can be seen as legacies from our past; not only our personal past, but from our relationships with parents, other family members, and through them, with our ancestors. Often these beliefs are only really challenged at times of transition, such as those we explored in lessons 1 and 2. The aim of psychosynthesis is to enable us to not be victims to these identifications, but to be free to choose. At all times of transition, particularly where you feel stuck or in pain and difficulty, it is worthwhile remembering to ask yourself: Is there some choice to be made in this transition?

It is the ability to make choices that enables us to become freer. This is to not say that identification and attachment is always or only negative. We have to identify ourselves so we can experience the world (whether through feelings, sensations or thoughts). Identification can be a rich source of pleasure. There is a great difference between a "chosen" identification, however, and those where we feel stuck, unable to make choices about what we want. The ability to both disidentify and re-identify enables us to feel stronger in our personal identity, to recognise ourselves, helps create order and have more choices available to us.

> Reflect: What do you currently believe about who you are? What are the beliefs you are holding on to about who you are? ...
>
> Which of these beliefs are you holding on to most strongly? With which beliefs about yourself are you most identified? ... [write]
>
> If you were to let go of any or all of these beliefs, what are you afraid of or might you be afraid of? ...
>
> Write a detailed argument AGAINST two or three of your most strongly held beliefs about yourself ... [write]

---- ¶ BREAK ----

The contents of consciousness

The experience of self-identification, of having an "I", is a particular feature of our human consciousness. This self-consciousness, however, is usually experienced, not simply as self-consciousness, but rather mixed with and veiled by the contents of our awareness, that is, everything we are sensing, feeling and/or thinking at any time. We usually live our lives identified with all this endless stream of consciousness. To fully experience self-consciousness, we need first to disidentify from the "contents" of consciousness.

As you have already seen, most people tend to be generally more attached to either their thoughts or their emotions, and can thus be described as mentally or emotionally identified. Such identification is useful at times, even necessary, but to live a balanced life we need to cultivate the spheres of experience in which we are deficient. People who are predominantly identified with their thoughts need to increase their awareness, experience and expression of their feelings, rather than diminish or decrease their mental awareness. Similarly, someone who is emotionally identified needs to investigate and refine their feelings while enlarging their connection to their mental side. In both these cases mind and feelings are unequally developed, and therefore of unequal size: the technique is to increase the size of the smaller one so that it matches the size of the larger one which you are working on clarifying.

Through deliberate disidentification from the personality and identification with the self, we gain freedom and the power to choose either attachment to or disattachment from any aspect of our personality, according to what is most appropriate for any given situation. Then we may learn to create an inclusive and harmonious synthesis in our whole personality.

An awareness meditation

The work of psychosynthesis is not about changing the content of the personality but changing our relationship to it, to become the you that has a personality rather than vice versa, then to realise that all personality issues are not about what you do but about who you are (beyond the content of your personality). The aim is to engender and continuously build a sense of the freedom to choose.

After preparation ... Ask yourself: What am I aware of? Continue asking this question, jotting down all the answers that come to you, either in a linear list or as spokes on a wheel. (Continue for at least 5 minutes.) ... [write]

After answering the question, reflect on how you felt while doing the meditation ...

Now ask yourself: Who am I aware of? Continue asking this question, jotting down all the answers that come to you, either in a linear list or as spokes on a wheel. (Continue for at least 5 minutes.) ... [write]

After answering the question, reflect on how you felt while doing the meditation ...

Now ask yourself: Who is aware? Continue asking this question, jotting down all the answers that come to you, either in a linear list or as spokes on a wheel. (Continue for at least 5 minutes.) ... [write]

After answering the question, reflect on how you felt while doing the meditation ...

Now reflect: Which of your subpersonalities have been involved in doing this exercise? ...

Which, if any, have not been involved? ... [write]

Who has the experience of having subpersonalities? ... [write]

¶ BREAK

Disidentification and self-identification

As far as we can tell, most if not all of the other creatures with whom we share our planet do not have a sense of self-consciousness. No dog will ever think: "I am me, myself, separate and different from everything and everyone else." This separate unique self is the simplest part or "unit" of our total being. It is our core. The self, understood in this way, is completely separate from everything else that makes us up—our bodies, feelings, thoughts, desires, all our subpersonalities, the different roles we play and so on. As it is separate, it is a place of unity and individual wholeness from where we can utilise and direct all these other elements that make us what we are.

And unlike these contents of our awareness, the self never changes, but remains that one static, unchanging, ever-present part of ourselves. One minute I am a father, then a lover, now I am feeling, then thinking—but I am always the self. The self is what makes us who we really are, separate not only from all the contents of our consciousness, but also from everyone and everything else too. As selves we each have our own individual experience. Of course, we might be identified and see ourselves as, say, a sportsman. This person might then become so identified with this role that he believes it is who he really is, rather than a role he is playing. Or someone might become so identified with their feelings they lose sight of the rest of their functions.

Thus, the great value of being able to disidentify from all these functions and roles and get to the true central core self. This self is not attached to anything so, if from this place you ask yourself: "who am I?" the answer is not a sportsman, a mother, a banker, an angry person, a thinker, a fool, an actor, or anything other than "I am me". Being identified is a bit like being in a dream where you move from one identification to another without awareness.

Some Eastern philosophies compare our waking "reality" to just such a dream. We don't realise we have, say, a particular feeling, we become the feeling. I don't have sadness, I am sadness. There's nothing wrong with that, per se, but such identification and attachment limits our perceptions. If we can awaken from this limiting dream, and identify with the self, we can come alive with a new awareness.

Let's posit that we have three states of consciousness: sleeping, dreaming and waking. Our ordinary everyday consciousness, when we are identified with something, is like dreaming, while being self-identified is being awake.

> Reflect: How do you know whether you are sleeping, dreaming or waking? ...
> Is there any way you could ever know? ... [write]

We often find it most difficult to disidentify from our thoughts. We construct our world through our thoughts about it, so it can feel dangerous or difficult to stop thinking about it. Maybe our world will fall apart and we will be left in an unstructured, undifferentiated state. In actuality, however, we find we are left with the self. We find a new clarity in our lives we never knew could exist before. Indeed, when we stop our inner dialogue with ourselves, we find that special and extraordinary aspects of ourselves are able to surface. We can make more creative choices about our lives, and more easily find ways to manifest these choices.

When we disidentify, we can then choose to re-identify. That is the goal. We don't want to be without our vehicles for expression and experience; we want to have them rather than them having us. It is as if when we re-identify with thoughts, feelings or the body, we can take a little bit of our new self-awareness with us. Not only have we found our "I", the self, and are more able to disattach ourselves from the contents of our consciousness, but also we can more effectively control our being and doing in the world in a positive, life-enhancing way.

From this new perspective, we can truly say "I am simply myself, and I have a body, and feelings and thoughts in order to experience the world and express myself in it." With this new strength, as well as being able to bring more clarity to what is happening in our lives, and having the ability to select what is the best choice for us, we also find we are generally happier and more effective in our relationships with other people. On top of this, we also then have an "safe anchor", so to speak, which allows us to more easily explore our lower unconscious and sort out some of the blocks, complexes, obsessions and other life-diminishing facets of our being. We have also, through this work, created more space for the influx of transpersonal energies into our personality. We are more able to manifest qualities such as Beauty, Trust, Joy, Truth and so on.

The benefits of disidentification, then identification with the self, cannot be over-stressed. You have already learned what is perhaps one of the simplest ways to start disidentifying from various roles. Through recognising subpersonalities, and naming them, you are separating yourself from these roles. If you can see, for instance, that part of you is, say, "a daughter", then you can realise you are not just a daughter. This applies to all our subpersonalities, whatever roles we play. It is perhaps more difficult to directly disidentify from the functions of thinking, feeling and sensing, but it can be done. It is achieved chiefly through a form of introspection whereby we become the "observer" of our life. We can look at everything that happens to us as distinct from ourselves. If we are angry, for example, we can step back, become an observer, and see our anger. Then we realise we are not our anger, rather anger is something we have.

We awaken from the dream, and see ourselves from a place of greater perspective. We might find it is right to be angry in the present circumstances, or not, but whichever is the case, we will have it rather than it having us.

The most important self-identification work we can do is through life situations as just described, when we observe ourselves from a separate place. As we do this more, we start to realise the truth that the self is a continuous presence behind all that happens in our life. It is always useful to forge links and strengthen our connection to the self, to help and foster this natural process. The exercise that follows helps us to do just that; it is the most important one in this book, and is central to the work of psychosynthesis.

¶ BREAK

The self-identification exercise

The following exercise is a tool for moving towards and realising the consciousness of the self.

Follow these instructions slowly and carefully:

> Relax yourself in the best way you know how, putting yourself in a comfortable but alert position. Take a few deep breaths, and let go of any tensions from the day so far. Follow the instructions slowly and carefully.
>
> Affirm to yourself the following: "I have a body and I am not only my body. My body may find itself in different conditions of health or sickness, it may be rested or tired, but that has nothing to do with my self, my real I. I value my body as my precious instrument of experience and action in the world. I treat it well, I seek to keep my body in good health, but it is not myself. As I am aware of having a body, I must be more than my body. I have a body and I am not only my body."
>
> Close your eyes, recall what this affirmation says, then focus your attention on the central concept: "I have a body and I am not only my body." Attempt to realise this as an experienced fact in your consciousness …

Now affirm to yourself: "I have feelings, and I am not only my feelings. My feelings and emotions are diversified, changing, and sometimes contradictory. They may swing from love to hatred, from calm to anger, from joy to sorrow, and yet my essence—my true nature—does not change. I remain. Though a wave of anger may temporarily submerge me, I know that in time it will pass, therefore I am not this anger. Since I can observe and understand my feelings, and can gradually learn to direct, utilise, and integrate them harmoniously, it is clear that they are not my self. I have feelings, and I am not only my feelings."

Close your eyes, recall what this affirmation says, then focus your attention on the central concept: "I have feelings and I am not only my feelings." Attempt to realise this as an experienced fact in your consciousness ...

Now affirm to yourself: "I have a mind and I am not only my mind. My mind is a valuable tool of discovery and expression, but it is not the essence of my being. Its contents are constantly changing as it embraces new ideas, knowledge and experience, and makes new connections. Sometimes my thoughts seem to be independent of me and if I try to control them, they seem to refuse to obey me. Therefore, my thoughts cannot be me, my self. My mind is an organ of knowledge in regard to both the outer and inner worlds, but it is not my self. I have a mind and I am not only my mind."

Close your eyes, recall what this affirmation says, then focus your attention on the central concept: "I have a mind and I am not only my mind." Attempt to realise this as an experienced fact in your consciousness ...

Now affirm to yourself: "I have a body, feelings and a mind but I am not only my body, feelings and mind."

Next comes the phase of identification. Affirm clearly and slowly to yourself: "After this disidentification of my self, the "I", from my body, my feelings, and my mind, I recognise and affirm that I am a centre of pure self-consciousness and of will, capable of observing, directing and utilising all my inner processes and my physical body."

Focus your attention on the central realisation: "I am I, a centre of pure self-consciousness and of will." Realise this as an experienced fact in your awareness ...

When you have practised this exercise a few times, you can use it in a much shorter form. The important point is to keep to the four main, central affirmations:

> I have a body and sensations, and I am not only my body and sensations.
> I have feelings and emotions, and I am not only my feelings and emotions.
> I have a mind and thoughts, and I am not only my mind and thoughts.
> I am I, a centre of pure self-consciousness and of will.

You may have to repeat the exercise a few times to start with to get its full flavour, but then you will be able to do it daily from memory. The effort will be well worth it. All the influences that try to capture your attention and demand identification will no longer have the same hold over you.

Perform the self-identification exercise at least eight times over a period of no more than two weeks, and keep a record of how you felt each time, and what results (if any) you may have noticed, directly after the exercise and throughout the following period. (There is no right or wrong response to this, trust your own.)

Some people find it difficult to follow the affirmations in this exercise that may seem to suggest that you are not your body, feelings or mind, objecting that this may cause a disassociation from these functions. A suggested alternative way of using the exercise, if this bothers you, is to change the disidentifying statements to "I have a body and I am more than my body; I have feelings and I am more than my feelings; I have a mind, and I am more than my mind." If you do this, it is important to always also affirm that you are more than all your body, feeling and mental experiences, focusing on the sense of being simply the "I" who has these functions.

¶ BREAK

Soul and the stages of life

The lessons now move towards including more of the "transpersonal" aspects of our psyche from where we can explore our developmental stages from a deeper, soulful perspective. It has been said that soul has

THE ART OF SELF-IDENTIFICATION 109

lessons to learn, experiences it needs to have, so incarnates and comes into the world with a clothing of body, feelings and thoughts in order to have these experiences. The soul is therefore evolving, it is in a state of process, having chosen to incarnate and live through this life to aid evolution. As personalities, we can either co-operate with this process or we can fight against it.

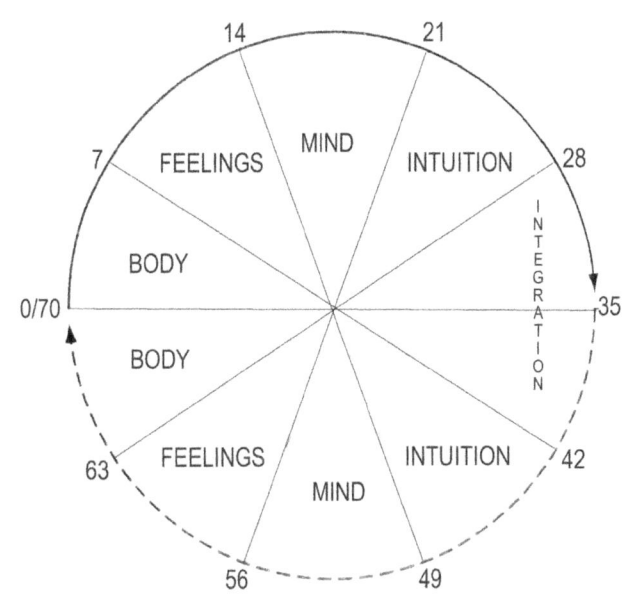

Diagram 6: The wheel of life

Diagram 6 illustrates how an average life of 70 years might be seen to have different emphases on growth depending upon which functions are forefront. Our physical, emotional and thinking functions develop from our birth onwards. Of course, these developments do not happen independently, but each seven-year period is shown as having one of the functions foremost for development. The others are also developing, but not in the foreground. Also, seven-year divisions are of course approximate averages, and not meant as rigidly defined age barriers. They present an overall picture, not the exact truth for any given individual.

So, keeping these limitations to the model in mind, uppermost for development from birth to around 7 years old is the body, which clearly agrees with our knowledge of the developing child. Of course, it must be stressed that other functions are developing through this period, it is simply suggesting that the body is currently foreground. Then during the ages from 7 to 14, emotional development is foreground (including the onset of puberty), from 14 to 21, intellectual development, and, from 21 to 28, intuitive faculties developing.

After that, the idea is that we are then working on integrating the different functions until we reach the second half of life. Working backwards, we can see that in the last seven years the physical becomes foreground again. Any issues not dealt with effectively in the first seven years are "repeated" or "brought up again" during this period. It is almost as if the soul creates a reprise, offering the individual the opportunity for further lesson learning and integration. For instance, in the last but one seven-year stage (if we were to take 70 years as the length of a life, then this is approximating between 56 and 63 years) there is a repeat of the emotional development period. Interestingly, this is an age where heart attacks are likely to happen. The ages from 49 to 56 relate then to mental development, and this is often the time when issues around life and meaning come to the fore.

To put the end of life at 70 is, of course, not accurate; people die at many different ages, and the average current age for people in the developed world is higher than that—though let's not forget that still in many parts of the world it is much less than that. This division of life into seven-year cycles is fairly artificial but it is representative of a process that occurs during life and gives us a model for the cycles of growth and integration we go through from a deeper perspective. Used in this way it can be most useful.

For a full, holistic development of your personality it is important to build your relationship with your thinking, feeling and sensing functions. This relationship is primarily developed through differentiation, and this model can sometimes help in orientating yourself. When something is happening, when you are experiencing or expressing something—anything—stop and ask yourself: what is this? Is this sensing, feeling or thinking? Be aware that you, as the "I" have these vehicles for experiencing and expressing yourself in life and now, as you identify more with the "I" rather than the contents of your consciousness, you can get a clearer picture of which of these functions are currently more or less foreground in your ongoing development. Without the "I", how would you have successfully achieved this?

Part of your task with psychosynthesis is to find ways to use the environment to support your work, rather than coming up against it.

As we discussed in an earlier lesson, if you are currently working on developing a more balanced relationship with your emotional function, for example, is it appropriate for you to go to that wild party tonight (it may be)? If your mental function needs development is a comic book the best reading material? Consider now: who makes the choice here, a subpersonality or you, the self, the independent, connected "I"?

You can purify and raise the level of each function to a higher vibration, continuously refining, so each function—body, feelings and thoughts—can become a clear channel for the expression of soul. Ask yourself questions like: What are the soul qualities trying to come through at this time? How can I evoke and develop these desired qualities? Would this be a good time to seek inner guidance? Shall I meditate on this now so that I am more aligned with my inner purpose?

---— ¶ BREAK ——---

Meditation

Many different meanings are given for the word meditation, and there are many different types of meditation and meditative techniques. At the simplest level, if we concentrate on something—anything at all—we are meditating. The more we discipline our thoughts, feelings and sensations to not intrude upon this concentration, the more deeply we can enter the meditative state. Many spiritual disciplines consider this work to be of prime importance. It is often imagined that meditation is primarily an abstract activity, involved with turning inwards and somehow transcending the "ordinary world". In fact, meditation does involve concentration, reflection, understanding, being receptive and so on. It also includes, however, ways of bringing these connections into outer expression, and it is thus also a very active and outer-directed technique. Meditation could be defined as the conscious and deliberate use of inner powers and energies to fulfil a specific purpose.

As a prerequisite to most types of meditation is to be able to still ourselves, the first action in meditation is to perform some acts that do this. We might slow our breathing down, sit in a particular posture, visualise a calming scene and so on. We have to shift our attention from its normal outward orientation towards the stillness of our inner world. To do this effectively, we can relax physically, enter a state of emotional peace and direct our thoughts to either stop or be one-pointed. Luckily for us, however, it is possible to meditate without achieving complete success in these preliminaries. The secret is to centre ourselves as best we can (perhaps through the self-identification exercise), and then simply trust that the wisdom of the self will lead us towards that with which we need to connect.

You have already been practising in your study of psychosynthesis a form of integrated meditation called reflective, receptive, creative meditation. To truly be able to receive, we need to firstly clear our minds of all our thoughts about whatever it is we wish to meditate upon. This is achieved in psychosynthesis by reflective meditation that, therefore, usually precedes receptive meditation. Then there would seem to be little point in connecting with the spiritual if we do not bring our new energy, connection and insights back to the mundane, material world, so to find ways to achieve this, psychosynthesis uses an expressive practice sometimes called creative meditation.

At times, of course, psychosynthesis uses many other forms of meditation, including contemplation, silent meditation, active meditation, one-pointed focusing and so on. Reflective, receptive and creative meditation is particularly effective, though, because it allows, if done in its entirety, for many levels of our being to operate and be active. Each of these three types of meditation can also be done singly, and often it is appropriate to do just that. If we combine the three together, however, it gives us the opportunity to meditate in a very thorough way that not only connects us to our inner being but also helps us express that connection in our everyday world. Both reflective and receptive meditation help us increase our spiritual awareness and thus deepen our ability to serve both ourselves and our fellow human beings. Indeed, all meditation is a form of service for as we make inner connections and express them outwardly, we increase the overall level of awareness in the collective consciousness.

The following exercise details how to do all three styles of meditation and to connect them together, grounding the resulting insights. It can easily be adapted to any subjects upon which you wish to meditate, or adapted to create different methods of meditation.

As said, the first requirement for meditation is to be able to relax. The most effective ways of relaxing and centring are ones you already know that work for you. It is usually helpful to choose as quiet a place as possible to meditate but, over time, you will likely build the ability to meditate even in a crowded room. It is usually preferable to sit rather than lie down, unless the exercise specifically asks you to lie. Choose a sitting position, either on the floor or in a chair, where you are upright but not rigid, your spine erect but not forced upright, and with your feet flat on the floor. For meditation, you might like to have your hands loosely clasped in your lap and have closed eyes. Before starting the meditative process take a few deep breaths and consciously choose to quieten your whole body.

<u>Reflective meditation</u>
Reflective meditation could be called "directed thinking". For this exercise I suggest you use a single word to focus your attention on your subject of investigation. The soul qualities such as, for example, Truth, Freedom, Justice, Beauty, Joy, Courage, Trust, Compassion, Peace, Loyalty and Patience, which we'll be exploring more in a future lesson, are a good place to start. You can, of course, use any other subject to meditate upon as is appropriate for your evolving process. For now, I'm choosing "Freedom" as the focus of the meditation.

Take a sheet of paper and put a circle in the middle with the word "Freedom" clearly written in it. Now quite simply think about this subject. Any words, images, ideas and so on that come to you as you think as one-pointedly as possible about this subject, put on lines radiating out from this circle ... [write]

When you feel you have exhausted your thoughts on the subject of "Freedom", continue for at least another five minutes. This allows you to delve deeper than you normally might, accessing deeper recesses of your mind. Your knowledge of the subject, through this kind of reflection, is stretched ... [write]

<u>Receptive meditation</u>
With receptive meditation, you tune into your unconscious and receive intuitions, inspirations, messages, energies and stimuli about your chosen subject. The most important requisite for receptive meditation is silence, as without it you cannot hear what your inner world is telling you.

Perform your receptive meditation in as quiet an external place as possible, and make your inner world as silent as possible also. Hold the concept of "Freedom" in your consciousness and try not to think of anything else. Be one-pointed in your determination to shut off all extraneous thoughts, feelings and sensations. Just be.

Do not do anything; just see what comes to you. Meditate in this receptive way for at least fifteen minutes …

Before continuing, record anything that came to you during this meditation … [write]

Creative meditation
Now consider what you have learned about "Freedom" from both your reflective and receptive meditations, and in particular how you could put this knowledge and understanding into action. Try to find which of these ideas are the most relevant to you in your life right now, then choose one item from your meditation that you would like to put into action.

Consider this one concept and find ways of acting upon it. Be precise and practical, so for instance, if you choose "to be more expressive" as the action, find ways to do this actively and practically. You might want to express your freedom very directly, or alternatively you might simply want to do something that requires more careful planning and execution. Even the simplest acts, rightly performed with intention, can be very effective.

———————————————— ¶ BREAK ————————————————

The mirror exercise

For this exercise you will need a mirror you can hold in your hand.

Sitting in a relaxed position, hold the mirror in front of you and ask yourself: Who do I see?

Continue asking yourself this question for five minutes, keeping your attention on the mirror. After the time is up …

Hold the mirror up once more and again ask yourself: Who do I see? …

Continue for a few minutes then, still looking in the mirror, ask yourself: Who is looking? Who is answering the question? …

Who is aware? … [write]

The "I" who is behind all the looking, all the content of your personality, is the "I" with which this type of practice helps us connect. This is a deeper sense of identity beyond all appearances, beyond all that we believe that we are. Often, we don't achieve such a rarefied sense of self, but the sort of exercises you have been doing in this lesson help you move to what in psychosynthesis is sometimes called "the clearest space available". This is an observer or director aspect of ourselves who is close to the "I". Remember, though, that the "I" itself is without any images or attributes.

It is best to consider the "I" as totally inclusive of everything, and not in any way as a disembodied thing, but rather as no THING at all. Then we can be awake, not so we can slip away from our earthly existence, but so we can come right on into it in our fullest being.

¶ BREAK

A wise being

We all have a source of wisdom and understanding that knows who we are, where we have been and where we are going. Our own "inner guide" is in tune with our unfolding purpose or true will and clearly senses the next step to be taken in the unfoldment of this purpose. As we contact it, we can better recognise the difficulties we are having in our growth and, with its help, can guide our awareness and will towards the resolution of these difficulties. Rightly used it can help us direct our energies towards achieving integration in our personality, and towards unifying the personality, soul and spirit into one living reality.

You can tell by the quality and tone of the "voice", which is never judgemental or prescriptive, whether it truly is this or just the chatter of your subpersonalities with their endless inner dialogue. Remember to check the validity of all messages. The more you are willing to confront and embrace your own way of working, the better able you will become able to discriminate between the inner dialogue and the true knowledge that emerges when the self-reflection is honest and deep enough. You are then learning to distinguish between what could be called "ego-insights" and "self-insights". While ego-insights are useful, particularly for making conscious links with the world, self-insights enable the recognition of the deeper Self within is not a separate entity but realised as a process of I–Thou relating.

There are many complicated rituals and procedures for contacting the "guardian angel" or "inner guide" inside yourself to assist your growth. The following procedure, however, is not only simple but also very effective.

> After preparation ... Take some time to let your body really become comfortable, but remain alert ...
>
> Close your eyes, take a few deep breaths and let appear in your imagination the face of a wise person whose eyes express great love for you ...
>
> Engage them in dialogue, and, in whatever way seems best, use the presence and guidance to help you understand better whatever questions, directions, choices, problems, etc., you are dealing with at this moment. This dialogue can be verbal or non-verbal, taking place on a visual and symbolic level of communication and understanding ...
>
> Spend as much time as you need with this wise person, then thank the image for having appeared to you, return to normal consciousness and write down what has happened ... [write]

You may not, particularly after some practice, need to actually imagine a person—they may be heard as a sort of inner voice, or even a direct "knowing" what is the best thing for you to be doing in any given situation. This wise being does not always have to be of the same gender each time they appear, or even to have a similar appearance. Images such as a flame, fountain or star, for instance, may appear, different images to meet the different needs at differing stages of your development and from which you can learn a lot.

You can adapt this simple procedure to dialogue with anything else, for example a part of your body. Try this: Have an inner dialogue with, say, your left hand and see what it has to tell you. Involve the hand in its external form, but also include its inner form, too—the bones, flesh and blood that all go to make the hand what it is.

If you find more detailed visualisation works well for you, you could create your own practice to meet your inner guide. For instance, you might start in a meadow, walk a path up a mountain (always taking your time with each stage and feeling anticipation growing within you), then at the top of the mountain meeting a wise person in a temple, engage them in dialogue, then, when completed, ensure you reverse the journey back to the meadow and ground yourself thoroughly.

Object attachment

> After preparation ... Choose three objects that are important to you—any objects will do so long as you feel attached to them. Take time with each object, reflecting on its importance and meaning in your life. Spend some time on this ...
> When you feel ready, consider now your attachment to these objects, not the objects themselves.
> What are you attached to? ...
> What would you lose if you no longer had these attachments? How do these attachments control or imprison you? ...
> And what would you gain if you no longer had these attachments? How do these attachments free you? ...
> (NB This does not say what would you lose or gain if you didn't have the objects, but if you did not have the attachments to them.)
> Regarding these attachments, what do you need to choose? ...
> Now reflect on the difference between an object and your attachment to it ... [write]

¶ BREAK

Before starting the next lesson

- Continue to stay in close touch with your sense of self. Practise the self-identification exercise regularly until you are very familiar with it, and able to comfortably use it when you wish.
- Consider: In my day-to-day life, what moves me towards or away from a sense of my true self? How do I know this?
- Give yourself at least one hour during which time you cannot be interrupted. Spend this time considering your experience of disidentification, self-identification and re-identification in light of what you've been exploring in this lesson.

LESSON 7

The power of imagination: living within the world we create

This lesson focuses on the significance of imagination and its transformative potential. Ancient philosophers claimed that imagination is superior to all nature and generation, and through it we are capable of being united to the gods, of transcending the mundane order, and of participating in universal life. Through imagination we are able to liberate ourselves from fate. In most esoteric traditions, the two forces considered to be central to all work are the will and imagination. This imagination clearly has little to do with idle daydreaming and unconnected fantasy.

The role of imagination extends to exploring the unconscious, fostering personal, interpersonal and transpersonal growth, and expressing inner wisdom in a stimulating way. It provides a connection to our inner world, where transformation is possible. This process may involve revisiting past experiences, reliving them to promote healing, and envisioning new, healthier narratives.

Images and symbols vary for each individual, and you are advised to find your own personal connections rather than relying on external interpretations. Then imagination can be harnessed for problem-solving, spiritual development and cultivating qualities like Joy. By understanding and integrating symbols, one can harness their transformative potential and promote personal and spiritual growth.

The lesson also continues to stress the importance of grounding mystical experiences, and reminds us that enlightenment is not a static state but a continuous journey. The principle of synthesis is highlighted as a way to balance opposites within us, fostering harmony and creativity. Ultimately, personal synthesis contributes to the growth of all sentient beings and moves the world closer to a universal synthesis.

¶ BREAK

Review

- Have you been regularly practising the self-identification exercise to familiarise yourself with it, and be able to comfortably practise it when you wish? If not, I strongly suggest you spend time on this now before continuing. It truly is the most powerful and meaningfully useful exercise.

Automatic drawing

Automatic drawing is a method of art-making in which the artist suppresses conscious control over the process, usually through one way or another of moving towards inner silence, then allowing the unconscious mind to do the drawing while the conscious choosing "artist" subpersonality is out of the way. The most famous artists using such techniques include Dalí, Masson, Miró and Bresson, artists mostly associated with Surrealism, but the methods go back at least as far as Da Vinci.

Who has not seen faces, animals, chariots and so on in clouds, and not only as a child, but such "vision" tends to get lost as we grow up, so part of the technique is to help you return to that pre-conditioned childhood state, even to before language formed your reality. The less you push for success consciously and leave it to the subconscious, the idea is that the more effective it will be.

A drawing is then done, allowing the pen to move automatically as if directed by the unconscious. Once completed, you can study it for information about the current state of your unconscious world.

For instance, you may reflect on its style—is it crowded, sparse, light, dark, freeing, oppressive, impersonal, regular, static or dynamic? What is the general atmosphere of the drawing like? Are figures, images, people emerging that mean something, which may represent different subpersonalities, for instance? Try free association, welcome intuitive flashes, be open to memories of past events that may be represented therein.

Then leave your drawing aside, let it sink into your unconscious and, if you want, after few days look at it again, inquire into its meaning for you, then let it go again. Then—put it away! Leave it several days before you come back to it to see how it now looks and what it may show you.

It's at this stage you can take it further and start to fill in the gaps to create an integrated drawing, but the technique works well even if you don't take it to this next stage. What an opportunity, though, it presents, as often the drawing reveals something specific—maybe a subpersonality, a relationship issue, the interface between the personal and transpersonal, and so on. Creating automatic drawings in this way is not only a matter of seeing something as something else but also the opposite, experiencing unity through diversity, ultimately the attainment of at-one-ness.

Use the following exercise to try this out for yourself—at the very least you can enjoy the sense of letting go and having something deeper inside yourself speak for itself.

For the following automatic drawing exercise, you may need coloured pencils and/or crayons later, and any other drawing implements you wish to use, but you can start simply with a pen or pencil. I suggest, if you can, to use the largest sheet of paper you have, but the practice works well even in small areas. Drawing in this way allows you the chance to be expressive without worrying about what you are going to express. If you have anxieties about drawing exercises, spend a little time focusing on what these are before beginning, and write a few notes about how you understand these anxieties.

> Before beginning, have a sheet of paper and a pencil or pen at hand.
>
> Pay particularly attention to relaxing and bringing yourself to centre yourself as usual. Take time to relax, and just be calm and aware ...
>
> Now let your hand do the drawing, don't think about it, or try and control it, just let the direction of the pen go wherever it does ...

straight bits, looping, curling, perhaps going into what seem like little drawings—even then, don't get caught up, just let it flow ...

Don't censor, judge or try to understand anything, let it come ... quick, flowing, twisty, straight, slow. Continue this free drawing for at least ten minutes ...

Try doing some drawing with the hand you don't usually use. Allow your expression free rein ... Continue for at least another ten minutes or more ...

When you have finished, look over the drawing and see what you can find in it. Are there symbols? Do parts of it look like something else? Can you see faces, animals, clouds, whatever? Look at the textures, lines, shapes, forms, colours, anything that catches your eye. It may be useful to fill in bits on the drawing at this stage, to make the things you see in it become more real. A cleverly placed eye, for instance, can make a face really come alive. Spend at least fifteen minutes on this process, preferably longer ...

Such drawing helps to mobilise your energy, breaks down old, unnecessary control, and is a means to express yourself. Free drawing can also be a dis-identifying experience if you really let yourself go with the pen. If it hasn't worked well this time, practise it more, perhaps with longer or deeper meditation before starting, or perhaps "just going for it" when you are moved to do so without any preliminary activities.

―――――――――――― ¶ BREAK ――――――――――――

About imagination

Imagination is our ability to form images or concepts of external objects that are not actually present to our senses, or are even non-existent. We can imagine a unicorn, for example, yet it is unlikely many of us have actually seen one! Imagination is thus the basis of the creative faculties of the mind. Anything that is created, whether artistically, scientifically or in any other way, is initially conceived of in imagination. In psychosynthesis, we use imagination to explore our unconscious, inner processes and to stimulate our personal, interpersonal and transpersonal growth. We also use imagination to express this inner learning and growth in our outer world in creative and life-enhancing ways.

Imagination offers us a symbolic connection to our unconscious, and can help us connect with all our unconscious processes. Once we make this connection, transformation is possible. Imagination can also help us to understand and express our inner wisdom in a stimulating way. Through using imagination to connect to our inner processes, we can bring underdeveloped parts of ourselves out into the open where they can gain independence. In fact, our imaginative faculties not only offer us a symbolic connection with our inner world, they can help us transform all our inner and outer relationships.

Although some images may be seen as universal, each one of us has our own world of imagery. To many of us today a white dove may symbolise peace, yet it may not only symbolise "food" but actually be an item of food to someone. In the West we may wear black to a funeral, yet in other parts of the world white may be worn. This is not to deny the importance of universal symbolism, which can be rich and rewarding to connect with. But it is of utmost importance that we find our own images and symbols inside and trust in our own inner processes. What something means to you has infinitely more meaning than any interpretation put on it by someone else. It is important to find your own imagery and find your own personal connection to symbols and myths.

When we start exploring the images that come up from our unconscious, it inevitably expands our awareness, but we need the will to do something about this awareness. If we do not integrate our increasing awareness, we run the risk of becoming "image junkies", always on the look-out for new images and symbols as if they were a drug feeding a false sense of "self", which inflates and separates us from any true connection to the transpersonal. On the other hand, if we do not explore the realms of imagery and symbols, but try to rely on what we already know, see and feel, then we run the equally dangerous risk of becoming rigid and sterile.

There are many ways to use the imagination. For example, in imagination we can try things out in a symbolic way. Both real and imaginary situations that frighten us can be accessed and worked on before the actual situation (for example, an interview) happens. We can use our imagination to change our relationship with different aspects of ourselves. Indeed, the many different ways of using our imagination to help us grow are only limited by the powers of our imagination. Anything we can imagine could possibly happen—and we can imagine just about anything.

Another use of imagery is to relive past experiences (whether "highs" or "lows"). If we allow ourselves to re-live a traumatic experience, for example, and fully experience the feelings, emotions and sensations that accompany the images associated with the experience, there is a possibility of transformation. When an old pattern is removed, we can make space for a new pattern. As several exercises in this course have already demonstrated, if you relive, through imagery, your early life experiences, for instance, and clear out some of the pain and difficulties associated with these experiences, you could then use images and symbols to recreate a "new birth" that is healthy and more life-enhancing. Such use of imagery, so long as it is genuinely accompanied by the associated experiences, can have a profound transformative effect on our personalities.

The power of the imagination is well known to advertisers, big business, politicians, and all those who would control or manipulate us in some way. If we see the same advertisement many times over and get bored with it and think the advertiser would do better to change it, then we are missing the point. Even if we consciously resist it, anything that is repeatedly presented to our senses has an effect. We may not think we bought a certain product as a result of advertising, yet in many cases we have done just that, albeit totally unconsciously. All images and symbols that we see or imagine tend to produce the physical conditions and external acts that correspond to them.

The fact that images repeated over and over sink into our unconscious, as it were, and affect us, can be used to our advantage. If we are affected by adverts in this way then we can choose to create our own adverts and respond to them. For instance, if you wanted to have more love in your life you might write a suitable affirmation on some cards—"I am worthy of love" perhaps—and place them around your house where you will frequently see them. You won't have to consciously look at these messages for, just like other adverts, they will work on an unconscious level. Then, if you become more worthy of love, it is quite likely you will get more of it.

> Consider the idea of self-advertising as described here, and what you could most usefully advertise to yourself. Create some cards, as suggested, and put them up at appropriate places in your home …
> After at least two or three weeks or so of having these adverts up, write a report on how, if at all, you feel they have affected you.

And don't be too quick to give up if you feel they haven't worked because, after all, this is an unconscious process. (This doesn't mean you cannot continue with the next section of this lesson before this time is completed.) ... [write]

--- ¶ BREAK ---

Manifesting and qualities

Through images, it is also possible to manifest positive qualities in your everyday life. If we used this power to contact, say, the quality of Joy and manifest more of it on to our planet it would be most positive. Symbols can help us discover and utilise our power, which can help us to choose what we want and reject what we do not want. In using our power in this way, we need to use our discriminative faculties to ensure we only manifest what is "for the highest good". When we truly own our power, and align ourselves through our sense of self with our purpose, we find we naturally discriminate with an easy inner wisdom.

We can use our imagination to manifest our power in many different ways. We can start, for example, with a given image, like the meadow or the mountain found in many of the exercises used in psychosynthesis. Sometimes we might just like to relax and let the images flow, trusting in the wisdom of our unconscious to bring up what is right for us at any given moment in time. Any way we choose to use images to aid our growth is effective if it comes naturally and is not forced. As our imagination is so rich, we need never force anything, but we do have to learn to trust in ourselves.

Real joy can be found in moulding the contents of the unconscious, controlling our inner world in a positive way, not so that we have "power over" anything or anyone, but so that we have "power with" the true nature of our inner being. When we start finding our inner freedom, when we are no longer controlled by images and fantasies but are able to use them for our own advantage, in an unselfish way, we are becoming psychologically mature.

All kinds of images, positive and negative, are continuously emerging from our unconscious. We can react to them or we can act upon them. In other words, we can have them or let them have us. If we have them then we can do what we want with them. We can feed upon the positive images, letting them grow bigger and stronger, and we can disperse the negative ones, not letting them take us over. For instance, we can quite simply take a positive image that is emerging from our unconscious, and consciously choose to make it grow bigger and bigger, letting it overwhelm us and fill us with its positive energy. On the other hand, when a negative image emerges from our unconscious, we can cause it to grow smaller and smaller until it disappears. We could even imagine it is totally consumed in the light of a burning, cleansing sun.

If we let ourselves go and trust in the emerging images from our unconscious, we can have a sense of being "new born" in that we are more able to connect with the "newness" of any situation without becoming identified or attached to what is happening.

> After preparation … Consider an image that is positive to you (trust whatever you think of, whether it is an obvious image or not). Make a note of, or draw a representation of this image so you can recall it …
>
> Now consider an image that is negative for you (again trusting what comes). Make a note of or draw a representation of this image …
>
> Sit or stand upright with your arms held out, your elbows bent, palms facing upwards as if you are holding two objects, one on each palm. Put the positive image on one hand and the negative image on the other (you can choose on which hand to put which image).
>
> Now imagine the positive image becomes bigger and bigger (and of course weightier and weightier) while the negative image becomes smaller and smaller until it shrivels up and disappears …
>
> It may take a little practice, but at some point, when the negative image disappears, the positive image will become so big (and heavy) you move your arms so that you are holding it in both hands. As this happens, bring this image into your body, and clasp both your hands over your chest or heart area …
>
> Stay with this for as long as you can, feeling the increasing energy from the positive image filling your being … [write]

———————— ¶ BREAK ————————

The essence of symbols

Symbols have been called the language of the unconscious, and when we start communicating with our inner world, we do so through symbols. To be truly understood and integrated, however, symbols cannot just be experienced on an intellectual level but must also arouse feelings and sensations. Neither can they be understood or interpreted out of context. A plane dropping bombs and a plane delivering needed supplies not only involve different concepts of "plane" (although the same plane can do both jobs) but also arouse totally different feelings. To truly understand a symbol, we have to get behind the outer form, which can veil and hide the inner meaning, and tune into the inner truth, the essence of the symbol.

In psychosynthesis, we are not so concerned with cold, rational analysis of symbols but rather choose to approach the essential inner form. Some of the ways of achieving this include:

- Simply considering the outermost form of the symbol, seeing what it shows you on its surface without any analysis or interpretation at all. It is often surprising and illuminating to discover that the symbols that emerge spontaneously from our unconscious often tell us so much just in themselves, without us needing to interpret or judge them in any way.
- Allowing the feelings and emotions that the symbol brings up to be fully experienced. Again, we can do this most effectively when we suspend judgement and interpretation. Feelings are truly about values, so when we allow ourselves to "feel" a symbol we discover its true value.
- Using our intellectual skills to discover what a symbol teaches us, penetrating into the deepest meaning of the symbol. Without having to rationally analyse a symbol we can use our thinking function to bring our knowledge into play and interpret the symbol in a clear and non-judgemental way.
- Letting the symbol's inner or deeper meaning intuitively emerge. Behind any of the sensations, feelings and thoughts we may have about any symbol is its more abstract, "bigger" meaning, an understanding that goes beyond our individual concepts about it. We cannot learn to be intuitive; we can only "let it happen". When it

does, we are then tuning into levels where we are more deeply in tune with the purpose of our soul.
- Identifying with the symbol, to discover the quality and purpose of a symbol. The form in which a symbol manifests may obscure its deepest meaning or it may not, but in either case, through identifying ourselves with the symbol we can start to connect with its deepest essence. To do this effectively we have to be centred and relaxed, and not attached to any of the thoughts, feelings or even intuitions we may already have about it. For example, you could do the self identification exercise and then consciously imagine you are the symbol under investigation. What then do you think, feel and sense?

We can change both our inner fantasy world and the outer "reality" on an individual and collective level. The symbols we need to work with never have to be suggested from outside, as our unconscious will invariably send us the right messages. When we can trust these messages from our inner world, we find they are transformative both to us as individuals and, through us, to our world as a whole. We can re-own symbols so they are part of the life-enhancing process of growth and evolution rather than leave them in the hands of those who would use them to control and manipulate others for their own selfish ends.

> Consider an image that has appeared to you in fantasy or dreams that has had a powerful effect on you. It may be somewhat abstract, but try to choose something as concrete as possible. Also, if possible, choose a strong image that has energy associated with it, either through the feelings or thoughts it evokes, through its recurrence in your life, or simply because it has some indefinably powerful effect on you.
>
> From what you have just read about approaching the deeper, inner meaning of a symbol or image, choose at least three of the five bulleted points above and use the techniques described to explore your image ... [write]

---------------- ¶ BREAK ----------------

The house of the self

When we use any kind of imagery, we are making a connection between the conscious and the unconscious. To make such a connection real in our everyday lives it is important to connect all these images with our body. We can also use our bodies as a source of symbols and images. How does your body feel at this moment? We can use the body as a starting place and then creatively use the images that emerge in our personal growth. In the following exercise, you will use your imagination to see your inner world in a concrete form.

> After preparation ... Make yourself comfortable, relax and centre. Imagine you are a house. See yourself as a house. What kind of house are you—a cottage, a terraced house, a grand mansion or what? Take some time to imagine what sort of house you are in as much detail as possible ...
>
> Picture this house in front of you and imagine you enter through the front door. This is no problem, for it is your house. You can explore the rest of the house some other time, but for now we will visit the basement or cellar ...
>
> Find the way down to the basement, and consider what it is like. Go into as much detail as you can, from assessing the condition of the foundations, the walls of the basement, the damp level, whether junk might be stored there, and so on. Assess whatever comes up so you get a good, clear picture of the full state of your basement. Really be as honest as if you were a surveyor checking the house for possible purchase ...
>
> Now recall it is your house and choose to do with it whatever you like. Change the basement in any way that seems suitable to you. Perhaps you need to reinforce the walls, or dry it out, or paint it, or throw away junk—take some time to make your basement into the sort of basement you would most like to have ...
>
> The power of your imagination will even allow you to add or remove rooms, completely change the shape or style of the basement, make of it what you will ...

If you relate the psychosynthesis egg diagram (see p. 33) to the house you have just imagined, it is quite easy to see how by exploring the basement in this way you have been exploring some aspects of your lower unconscious. At other times you can explore other parts of the "house", including "going upstairs" to examine your superconscious. Remember, however, that whatever you may find upstairs or downstairs, it is most useful when you bring it into your everyday life, the "living room" of your house, and use it in a way that assists your growth and development. What did you discover in your basement that it would be useful for you to bring up to the living room and utilise in some way?

¶ BREAK

The spirit of synthesis

Just as in an earlier lesson we saw that psychosynthesis comes alive and reaches some of its most meaningful insights when it is applied to relationships between individuals, psychosynthesis can have a vital part to play in the totality of interdependence between all living creatures. No one really exists as an isolated individual, anyway, for we all have involved and intimate relationships with other people and beings and our world in general, and thus we are truly interdependent. If we look at the whole of life in this way, we can see the potential, at least, for one family of living beings that co-exists harmoniously within itself and within the world it inhabits. On a spiritual level we can imagine the transpersonal Self as that which includes all the individual parts that make up the collective totality of existence and which is beyond each individual part. It is a general principle of synthesis that the whole is greater than the sum of the parts.

If four people stand around a heavy object and they try to lift it into the air they may manage it, but there is a lot of effort involved and the whole procedure will appear clumsy and uncoordinated. If before they try to lift the weight they breathe together, matching their breathing to a common cycle, then they count from one to ten together and all lift at the same moment, they will find the weight is remarkably easy to lift.

There is nothing strangely mystical or magical about this. The four people trying to lift the object together but in an uncoordinated way have the sum of the lifting capacity of all four of them minus what they lose through not being synthesised into one "lifting unit". If they perform acts to bring their action together then they become "a whole that is greater than the sum of the parts". The lifting becomes easier, and, you will find if you try this with some friends, is accompanied by the release of much energy. What was an effort before is transformed into a pleasure.

We all form groups like this to perform our various tasks in life. These groups include our family, groups we form locally where we live for various purposes, our work groups, social classes, unions of various kinds, our national groups, and so on through the group we call the entire human family to the group that includes all living beings. If we can apply this principle of synthesis to all these groups to which we belong, then we find that the tasks become easier and there is a release of positive energy, which can be used not only for the good of the group involved but also for other associated groups as well.

It is rarely that simply, however. Problems arise between individuals within groups and between groups that are not dissimilar to the problems that arise within the individual. As you know, as individuals we are composed of many different subpersonalities, and the people in any group can be compared to subpersonalities. The methods and techniques used in psychosynthesis to harmonise the inner world can be well applied to the outer world, too. Indeed, the drive towards unity we feel inside when we touch into the deepest aspects of our nature can be seen and applied to outer groups and situations as well. When we make this connection, we start to realise that the Self creates diversity from unity in order that all beings can find their own way to realise the unity from whence they came and to which they are returning.

We have the opportunity from a place of division to form a union, to come together with another being and be at one with them, or even to come together with all other beings and realise a total union. Without the division no such knowledge would be possible. While we are in this illusion of duality, however, we can help bring more beauty and harmony into the world through our clear consciousness of loving what we do and doing what we love. Then we help move the whole of life towards that final goal, the supreme synthesis where all the parts of life come together and realise the whole that includes all and yet transcends each individual part.

It is important to stress here that this is not an ungrounded, "mystical" view of life or of the place of individuals within the unfoldment of the universe. Of course, no one would want to deny the reality of a mystical experience that separates an individual from their mundane, earthly existence and, in a state of bliss, leads them to temporarily forget all outer reality and the environment. If we become attached to such experiences, however, we fall into the mystical trap. Psychosynthesis stresses the importance of avoiding this through always paying attention to bringing all transpersonal energies back to ground and finding a way of expressing them in the "ordinary world".

The mystical experience should not be seen as an end in itself but rather a step along the way from which the individual who has the fortune to have such an experience can draw creative energy and enthusiasm. The true mystical experience also brings with it the desire to come back into the world to express the energies involved and help one's fellow human beings to also experience this enlightenment. The "mystic" who remains spaced out has missed the boat, as it were, that carries us all, irrespective of our experiences, towards the final goal of fully realised and consciously shared unity.

The other mystical trap is to believe that once one has reached some sort of blissful state, or received some sense of enlightenment, that this is all there is to it. It is the experience of all the great mystics that enlightenment is neither an end in itself nor, as such, does it last forever. Nothing remains the same, everything changes, and the enlightened state is no exception to this cosmic rule. Everything that is alive is in a constant state of movement, constantly renewing itself as it moves from moment to moment. If you stop moving, quite simply you die but, even then, this is an illusion for in death we may find at the very least decay and a return to an energy state and perhaps more. Each revelation has to be grounded and expressed and also not clung to. The true mystic is the one who is working to express the energies with which they have connected, not the one who remains connected and has nothing left to say, do or feel.

> Reflect: How much work do I put into expressing the energies with which I connect? ... [write]

¶ BREAK

Synthesis—an organic process

It is worth stressing the principle of synthesis: that the whole is greater than the sum of the parts. If we look at a painting and analyse it into its component parts we may find the different colours, brush strokes, shading and light, figures and background—we may even find beautiful scenes depicted within it, trees, people, places—but we have to see it as a whole, in its entirety before we can realise the value of it as a great work of art. What comes out of that synthesised whole is something beyond any or all of the individual components, perhaps something that even transcends the artist's original conception.

In the psychological application of this principle of synthesis, we stress the importance of each part being made whole in itself before it can be truly synthesised with other parts. If one of your subpersonalities is not "whole", if it has wants at odds with your true purpose, if it has unheard and unmet needs, if its true qualities are obscured, then how can it take its true place as part of the whole personality without creating disharmony? It is so important, therefore, that we do not short-change our work on the personality, which is, after all, the "vessel" through which we express our innermost spiritual truths.

Synthesis is, in fact, an organic process. We cannot force it or make it happen, but what we can do is co-operate with and facilitate the process as it organically unfolds. One way of achieving a move towards actualising this potential that we all have is to work at balancing and synthesising the opposites that exist within us. If you identify as a man then you can work at bringing out the "female" within you to create more harmony and balance. If you are an idealist then perhaps you need some practicality to help balance your personality. If you are attached to the spiritual path then perhaps a little sensuality may lighten your load. Each of us as individuals has our own inner connection, our own inner world of opposites. The work of synthesis, in this area, is to find these opposites within ourselves so that we can balance them and create a clearer synthesis.

A further principle of synthesis is that we can never solve a problem at its own level. If we take the example of two subpersonalities who are in disagreement, perhaps about whether we should take a certain decision in life, then so long as we remain on the level of their argument it will continue. Both the parts are fighting for their rights, even for their very survival. Each part knows what is best for us and is going to "damn-well" make sure we do just that. If we can gain a perspective from a different level, however, we may be able to find a way to overcome the difficulty. One part of you wants to go out right now and another part wants to stay in. From a third place of greater perspective, we might find that a compromise can be reached—you'll stay in now but go out later, for example.

Once we have disidentified from both of the parts in this way, we have moved ourselves, if not actually to the place of the self, at least to a clearer space. We are no longer caught in the problem at its own level. Once we are thus placed, we can then start looking for a synthesis, perhaps through asking ourselves what it would be like if the two parts not only found a compromise but actually came together. We can do this at least partly through not being too attached to fulfilling the individual wants of each part but looking towards finding out what their real needs are. When we do this, we are moving these parts a little towards unity, towards the synthesising centre that is the Self.

Such a synthesis is not only possible, it is desirable. We can be both loving and strong, intuitive and logical, spontaneous and disciplined, idealistic and practical, spiritual and sensual, and so on. Indeed, what we usually find is that when we start bringing opposites together, we again get a sense of the whole that is greater than the sum of the parts. A new reality is created. I am still loving but now I can be strong when it is necessary and not allow people to just walk all over me, taking advantage of my good nature. I can still be a spiritual person and can better express my connection to the transpersonal not in spite of but because of my new connection to the world of the senses.

When we create synthesis in our lives, when parts within us come together into a new relationship, or when we find a way of moving closer to someone or something else in this true synthesising manner, then we not only grow individually, we add to the total growth of all sentient beings. We also free up energy that was previously blocked and involved in conflict, energy we can then put to creative uses. The more we move towards our personal synthesis, the closer we move the whole of creation towards the time when there is a universal synthesis.

> Reflect further on what you have just read and consider how can you apply what you learn in your life? ... [write]

--- ¶ BREAK ---

Are you you?

There are many stories that come from the Middle East that involve an imaginary foolish wise man called Mulla Nasruddin. Here is one such story.

Realising that he had forgotten who he was, the Mulla rushed through the streets, looking for someone who might recognise him. The Mulla rushed into a shop and demanded of the shopkeeper: "Did you see me come into your shop?"

"Yes, I did," replied the shopkeeper.

"Good. Now, have you ever seen me before?"

"No."

"Then how do you know it is me?"

> Reflect on this story before continuing. What is it about for you? ...
>
> Now reflect: How do you know you are you? ...
>
> Take care. The question is not how do you know who you are, but how do you know you are you!
>
> Use your physical form, gestures and dance to express your sense of the "you" you are ... [write]

---¶ BREAK---

Before starting the next lesson

- What do you imagine is the most useful or meaningful exercise you could perform while studying the power of imagination? Create and write out this exercise in detail ...

Perform your exercise!

- Give yourself at least one hour during which time you cannot be interrupted. Spend this time considering your connection and use of your imaginative faculties in light of what you've been exploring in this lesson.

LESSON 8

Purpose and the process of willing: personal and spiritual empowerment

Lesson 8 takes a deep dive into the concept of the will, exploring various stages and aspects of how the will operates. It begins by discussing the will as an essential but often elusive part of our decision-making process. It reflects on how we sometimes fail to act on our will, leading to feelings of guilt or shame. The importance of understanding where our choices originate is emphasised and how our subpersonalities influence our decisions. The idea of aligning our personal will with a higher, transpersonal will to realise our true potential and freedom is highlighted.

The stages of will are divided into four phases: "having no will", "knowing that will exists", "having a will", and "being will". As you progress through these stages, you move from feeling like a victim of circumstance to becoming the director of your own life, aligned with your innermost purpose. Having this deeper, connected understanding of how the will operates enables us to connect to "good will", which combines the energies of love and will. Acts of good will are dynamic and promote understanding and cooperation.

Lastly, the lesson touches upon the idea of freedom, distinguishing between freedom from past conditioning and freedom for the pursuit of positive goals. The source of the will is the place where true freedom arises, a silent inner place beyond the distractions of the world.

In practical terms, the lesson suggests exercises to strengthen both the strong and the skilful will and to promote the good will, self-reflection on one's purpose, and deepening one's connection to the source of will through connecting deeply to inner silence, always referring these practices back to your own grounded life experiences.

Review

- Did you create an exercise or practice using the power of imagination, and did you try it out?
- Did you give yourself at least one uninterrupted hour considering how you use your imaginative faculties?
- Have you been regularly practising the self-identification exercise to familiarise yourself with it, and be able to comfortably practise it when you wish? You are really strongly recommended to continue practising self-identification frequently.

The act of will

The will (or perhaps more properly "the process of willing") is the inner force that is available to each individual for the actualisation of their potential. Assagioli regarded the will as the central element and direct expression of the "I" or "self". He liked to use the analogy of the will as being like the helmsman guiding a ship, providing the direction rather than the power for moving the vessel forward.

Simply put, every choice or decision we make is an act of will. Consciously connecting with the dynamic energy of the will gives us the ability to be, to do and to become whatever we wish. All aspects of the will can be enhanced with training and practice. Once we use our will, it enables us to use our will further. It is inevitable, however, that obstacles will appear to block this development. Our awareness may become clouded or our attention diverted; we may feel overwhelmed and incapacitated. Working with the will may not be easy, but its rewards can be stupendous. Through the skilful use of the will, complemented by love, each individual has the potential to actualise them.

Reflect on how you use your will. How successful are you in using your will? Be honest but not judgemental of yourself ...

Who chooses in your life? ... [write]

---¶ BREAK---

Making a decision

This exercise is in two parts, with a break between. Make sure you do take the break.

Remember a time, an experience when you felt you were on track with your will and expressed yourself successfully, a time when you felt you successfully willed ...

As much as you can, make that experience alive for you now. Really enter into it. Remember where you were, what you were doing, what was going on ... What were you wearing, thinking, feeling? Was anyone else involved? ...

See if you can tune into or extract from that experience what the essence or quality of it was. What made the act of will successful? What would it be like to bring that essence or quality into your life now? ... [write]

---¶ BREAK---

Not making a decision

Remember a time, an experience when you knew it was right to make a decision, a certain choice, beyond a shadow of a doubt, a time when it was certain, you knew you had to do something and you didn't do it ...

How did you stop yourself? Be aware of how it was you didn't do it, however it was ...

What was the process you went through that led you to not doing it? What was it like for you afterwards? What did you feel after you didn't do it? ... [write]

The will exists whether we act upon it or not. When we don't act on it and it concerns something we know is important to us, we may feel guilt, shame, or a sense of betraying ourselves. We might try to cover it up, regain control of ourselves and pretend it never happened. We may create rationalisations and justifications to try to absolve ourselves of the bad feelings.

> What procedures did you go through to try to disguise or deny your feelings at the time in question? ...
> Would anything be different if you could make that choice again? ... [write]

It is important to consider what you are identified with in your life and the consequences to you of that identification. Whatever you have been connecting with in the last exercise, ask yourself:

> Who has been saying these things? Who is using my will? It may be a judgemental part of yourself, or an inner parent, an achiever, a pleaser, a rebel, or some other part of you ...
> Now ask yourself: Where were the choices coming from? ... [write]

It is said that the will is a natural process, an experience that cannot be described adequately with words, the spark of the self, the central mystery of life, something that precedes consciousness. However, it is possible to distinguish the source of the will itself from how it manifests in the personality. It is only by making such distinctions, and finding ways to align the personal will with the transpersonal will, that we realise our true potential through our freedom to choose.

―――――――――― ¶ BREAK ――――――――――

How will works

Every choice or decision we make is an act of will. We might not be aware that we have chosen, and may even feel like a total victim with no choice at all. Nevertheless, wherever we are and whatever we are doing, it is our choice. Without making a choice, we could not stay where we are or move anywhere else. Without making a choice, we could neither stop what we are doing nor continue doing it. Every time we make a choice, we perform an act of will. We have many different inner powers, and the right use of these powers can enable us to make the best choices both for our own well-being and the world around us. We can only make these choices, however, through developing these inner powers in a balanced and conscious way.

The discovery of our will and its subsequent training can be best achieved through direct experience. If we make a comparison with a car, the first thing we have to learn is that there is an engine through which we can choose to move the car. Then we have to find ways of using that engine so that we can travel in the direction that is best for us at any given moment.

Of course, a lot of the time our actual experience is very different from this. Even if we are aware we have a car, it certainly doesn't feel like we are in the driving seat! We are drifting or muddling along as if we are the victims of our circumstances. We see ourselves as the victims of where we are or who we are, of poverty or depression, of failure or even success! We are the victims of other people who made us whatever we are, or stop us doing what we wish. We feel as if we are not really free to choose what we want. Since childhood we have been told by parents and teachers and other "well-wishers" that we need to face the "reality" of life. The message, that we cannot have everything we want, easily becomes one that says we cannot have anything we want.

If someone asks us to do something, the two obvious responses are yes and no. We can say we will or we will not. Yet, usually, we have a third choice available to us: "not for now". We do not have to limit ourselves by saying yes or no when "not for now" is more appropriate. Sometimes it is right to make quick and immediate responses. The question at hand needs a fast response, or it is so obvious which choice is needed. Often, however, we can take the time to consider our choices and make them in a more centred, balanced way. The more consciousness we bring into our decisions, the more we are able to choose what are the right decisions for us.

Any act of will actually takes place through six distinct but, in practice, interwoven steps:

- investigation (finding out what it is we wish to do);
- deliberation (considering all the different things we wish to do at any time and selecting the acts most relevant to our current situation);

- decision (deciding upon the one act that is most important to us at the present time, and clearly formulating and stating this desire);
- affirmation (staying connected to this decision through constantly reaffirming that this choice is what we really desire to achieve);
- planning (thinking about the different ways we can actually make whatever it is happen);
- execution (doing it, finding ways of carrying out the intended plan, either in entirety or step by step).

Every choice we make involves these six steps to a greater or lesser degree. It might be that for a particular choice we know what we want, hardly have to deliberate over it at all, and are able to quickly plan and execute the action necessary to succeed. For example, a choice to go to a nearby shop to purchase something we need. On the other hand, we might not really know what we want, and we might endlessly deliberate over the choices and never actually decide what to do. Or we might know exactly what we want and yet not know how to go about planning and executing the necessary actions. Our desire could be something well worked out, but for which the execution needs to take place at a particular time. If we choose a sunset, we will only be able to "make it happen" at the right time of day.

While our acts of will always include all the six steps, they rarely do so in a linear fashion. For instance, while planning we may need to go back and deliberate further when we discover that we have not quite got the choice right. Often, we need to keep going back to our choice to affirm it over and over. Constantly returning to the affirmation step to focus on and strengthen our choices is usually a good technique as it reinforces the planning and execution of our desire.

We also have to consider that every choice we make affects everything and everyone else. If I choose to eat this particular orange right now, I will never be able to eat it either now or at any other time. That may not seem so serious, as, after all, there are plenty more oranges. In other circumstances, however, such knowledge takes on much more significance. For example, someone may choose to ignore their knowledge that a diesel car is damaging to the environment. That they continue running such a vehicle may seem to make no difference, because after all what difference can one person make? Yet in reality the situation will surely be worsening.

We must make our choices clearly and with heart, and be aware of this global effect, yet we must not allow such knowledge to make us impotent. Rather we must try to align ourselves with the flow of nature so that our choices add to rather than subtract from the evolution of consciousness on our planet.

> Consider the six steps involved in the act of will just as described: investigation; deliberation; decision; affirmation; planning; execution.
> Select something you wish to achieve in your life, whether it is something relatively major (for instance, changing your occupation) or something relatively minor (for instance, buying a book). Whatever you choose, consider how you can go about achieving this using the six steps of the will ... [write]
> If it is possible, do it! If not, consider why not: There may be practical reasons, or there may be internal blocks and resistances to whatever it is you have chosen ... [write]

---------------- ¶ BREAK ----------------

The stages of willing (1)

It is important to understand the distinction between the steps, as just described, in making an act of will, and the different stages we go through in developing our connection to will. Although the process is, in actuality, continuous, as individuals we can experience the will as having four stages. The first stage could be described as "having no will". It is a common human experience to feel like a victim to outside forces, other people or the circumstances in which we find ourselves. At many times in our lives, we all experience a sense of impotency, frustration and an inability to act. Instead of doing what we wish, we become totally reactive to the circumstances or the environment. We feel as if what we are, and what we are able to do or not do, is totally dependent upon what happens outside of us.

At these times we act like a victim to our repressed urges and desires, to basic drives, or to people or events outside of us. When we are coming from this state, when we believe ourselves to be "will-less", our primary motivation is desire. We do not see ourselves as having any control, but instead experience ourselves as "slaves of desire", whether we are fully conscious of this or not. Our one wish is to get our desires met and to avoid as much struggle, effort and pain as possible. If we have to manipulate people we will so long as our desires are met. As we reduce our responsibility in this way, we become even more a victim and we can easily sink further into this deadening trap.

In reality, however horrible the situation you are in may truly be, you can make of it what you will. You could be unjustly imprisoned and, as a victim, spend your days bemoaning your fate. You might plot revenge on those who unjustly imprisoned you, those to whom you are a victim. Or you could undertake some other plan of action—you could meditate, write, use the time to make detailed observations of yourself or your fellow inmates, and so on. There are many stories of people doing just this. Assagioli, when imprisoned by Mussolini, spent his days developing his system of psychology by exploring what lessons he could learn from fellow prisoners. In other words, Assagioli, in this unjust situation, chose to take responsibility for himself and not sink into a victim role.

Of course, we do not have to be in such an extreme situation to feel like a victim. Think of times right now when you feel like a victim. Perhaps you are a victim to your boss at work, or to your partner, your parents, or even your children! Perhaps you feel like you are a victim to the unjust society in which you live. The key to releasing yourself from this victim consciousness is to realise that, whatever is happening to you, you are creating the situation. We all re-create our worlds afresh each and every moment.

> Reflect: Who is running your life? Are you directing your life? Are you free? Are you in control of your life? ...
>
> To what extent do you feel a victim (be truthful)? To what extent do you feel a victim to other people? ... to circumstances? ... To what extent is the direction of your life determined by outer events? ... [write]

---— ¶ BREAK ———

The stages of willing (2)

The next stage of the will process is coming to an understanding that "will exists". We might still feel we cannot actually do it, but we know, whatever it is, that it is possible. We realise we have a choice. This choice in any situation is always, as we have already discussed, "yes", "no", or "not for now". Of course, we may have reached this stage with a part of our personality but be less developed in other parts. Even if this stage of the will is only partially experienced, however, it leads to a shift in awareness from unconscious desires to active, conscious wishes. We might still feel separate, but there is a beginning of responsibility, the knowledge that some choice is possible. We are starting to develop our personal power.

Once we know that the will exists, we are able to start working on developing it within ourselves. There are two basic aspects of will power that we can develop and, in psychosynthesis, we call these "the strong will" and "the skilful will". Strong will is the energy to choose while skilful will is the knowledge of how to use that energy. The strong will is like a car, the skilful will the driver. We can learn to develop both strong and skilful will. In most of us, one will be developed more than the other, but there is usually room for improvement in both.

One of the best ways to develop the strong will is to find ways in your daily life of being strong willed. You may hate washing up, for instance, so to develop your will you could choose to do it regularly and with positive attention. You could choose to make physical acts into acts of will. If you were gardening, for instance, you could do it consciously, being aware that each spade full of earth you move, or each flower you plant is an act of will. You might do aerobic exercises, or dancing, and do this not so much just for the exercise value, but because each movement you make you are consciously choosing to make. You could choose to read stories or watch YouTube videos about great heroic deeds performed against all odds. You can easily devise other techniques for strengthening the strong will, but above all perform these techniques playfully, cheerfully and with interest.

You can also develop skilful will through acts in your daily life. When washing up, for example, you might ask yourself what is the most skilful way to do this, to make it most efficient and with the least expenditure of unnecessary energy. Should you wash the greasy pans or the glasses first? The development of skill is accomplished not only through what you actually do but through the attitude you have to the act being performed. It's not what you do, it's how you do it. Part of this skill is being aware of how much energy you put into doing something. If you put in too little energy, it's like using a spoon to move a mountain; using too much energy, it's like taking a forklift truck to an egg!

To develop strong will you can:

- do selective reading, choosing to read books—either fiction or non-fiction—that encourage this, stories of great heroic deeds against all odds, books about "getting what you want" and so on;
- perform useless will exercises; for example, taking all the matches out of a matchbox, counting them carefully and deliberately, one by one, as you do so, then reversing the procedure. This is comparable to the exercises an athlete might perform, in themselves of no value, but all part of strengthening your ability to perform when required;
- find ways in your daily life of being strong willed; for example, if you hate washing up you can choose to do it regularly and with positive attention;
- score successes and failures; keep a score card of your acts of will, those that come off and those that don't and strive to improve your performance and score;
- make each physical act an act of will—a tall order, but you could, say, when gardening, do it consciously, bringing awareness to your acts. Or perhaps choose to do exercise, or dancing, and be aware that all your movements happen because you choose to make them happen.

You can easily devise other techniques for strengthening the strong will, but above all perform all these techniques playfully, cheerfully and with interest.

To develop skilful will you can:

- find the most skilful way to do something, to make it most efficient and with the least expenditure of unnecessary energy. The development of skill is accomplished not only through what you actually do but through the attitude you have to the act being performed. It's not what you do, it's how you do it;
- be aware of how much you put into doing something, making it a conscious choice to use the necessary energy for the job but not over- or under-do it;
- most importantly do self-identification exercises and create a strong contact with your "I", your centre of consciousness, and take decisions from this centred place. The greatest skill is making the most appropriate choices, and you can do this most effectively when you are not identified.

Choose at least one way you can work on developing your strong will, and another way to develop your skilful will. You might use the examples given above, or create your own ways of doing this. Spend at least six days working on these techniques you choose, refining their application and noting what resistances emerge within you ... [write]

--- ¶ BREAK ---

The stages of willing (3) and (4)

Once we have developed our will, at least to some degree, we pass to the next stage of the will, which in psychosynthesis we call "having a will". When this stage or level is attained, it can be experienced consciously or unconsciously, but it happens, usually, through a gradual awakening. We start to become a "director" in our life. When we have chosen to play a particular role, we hold both an awareness of the self or centre, and the role that we are playing. We switch between them as appropriate.

At this stage of the will, that is when we consciously realise that not only does the will exist but we have a will. This engenders a distinct move towards integration where there is less fragmentation and more clarity of choice. We realise that we have a will and we can choose with it. We start to feel more connected to our purpose for being alive on this planet at this time. From this place we truly take responsibility for our acts. Of course, we may not be responsible and conscious in this way all of the time, but the amount of time we spend in this state gradually starts to increase.

The fourth and final stage of the evolution of the will in the individual is called "being will". When this stage is reached there is alignment with the transpersonal Self and the deepest, most spiritual aspects of will. We are connected with our innermost understanding. We can reach this level of consciousness through meditation, through silence, or simply through turning inwards and allowing this energy of the Self to permeate through us. Once we have reached this stage, even for a moment, it is inevitable that we will desire to express this deep and meaningful connection in the outside world. Indeed, it is the sign of true "spiritual attainment" not when the person involved can sit for hours in a yoga posture, or perform "miraculous" feats, but rather when this energy is expressed in the world in a way that brings healing and sustenance to his or her fellow beings.

When we start using our will from a centred place, we find we are the source or cause of what happens in our life and are not just an effect or victim to circumstances. We discover there is a distinction between our "true will" or purpose, which can be defined as the will of the Self, and the energies, such as drives and self-centred desires, that come from subpersonalities. Of course, this is not to say that subpersonalities should not get what they want—their needs have to be met fully before they can truly be transformed. But their wishes are inevitably in conflict with the wishes of other subpersonalities. We experience no such conflicts with the "true will" for this originates from the deepest, innermost core of our being. Indeed, one way of knowing it is "true will" is the total lack of conflict experienced.

We can only truly discover our true will or purpose when we consciously and actively take steps towards its manifestation. That may seem obvious, but too often we forget this and, instead of following our path a step at a time, we try to leap ahead, not paying attention to what is happening in the present moment. As was stressed in previous lessons, the next step is always of utmost importance, and, in actuality, the only step we can make. Even physically if we try to take more than one step at once we are more likely to fall over than succeed. This is even truer when we are talking about inner purpose. We find it is easier to stay on our path if we pay attention to our immediate position, rather than worrying about something way ahead.

We may have little or no idea of what our true will is, but if we reflect upon what purpose means to us, and what we would like to manifest in our lives that has "real meaning", we can start getting at least an inkling of it. You might like to try some reflective, receptive and creative meditation on "purpose". Remember that purpose always follows the rule of non-interference—it cannot be your real purpose if it involves you interfering with or altering someone else's purpose.

When we have connected to our purpose through meditation as suggested above, or through any of the other methods used in psychosynthesis or other ways to self-realisation, the next step is to decide how to manifest purpose. The techniques for grounding that we have already discussed can be most helpful in this, but the most important thing is to find your own individual ways of manifesting your purpose. This is where it is often most helpful to have a good guide who will be able to not only help you connect with your purpose but also help you to find ways to manifest it.

> Reflect: Do you have purpose in your life? What is it (or what might it be) and how does it (or can it) manifest in your life? ... [write]

--- ¶ BREAK ---

Willing from the heart

The will is not only active, not only involved with "doing". You could choose, for example, to just be, to pass some time doing nothing. One of the greatest distortions in our thinking about will power is to believe it has to be an effort, or that it depletes our energy in some way. On the contrary, when we make conscious, definite acts of will rather than ending up with less energy, we feel energised, more alive, more present in the world.

We need to be flexible and be able to find a balance between active and passive acts of will. Both can require strong and skilful will. To say "no" to something, for instance, might require a tremendous act of courage if friends are encouraging you to do it. Or to exhibit patience in waiting for something you madly desire can require great reserves of strong will. The more centred we become, the more able are we to make acts of will, either active, passive, strong or skilful, as the situation requires.

One result of moving towards our centre and making our acts of will more conscious and purposeful is that we find there is another aspect of the will, sometimes called "the good will". Acts of will that are made from the heart, that are filled with sympathy, love, understanding and warmth, are all manifestations of the good will. When we have good will towards someone, whether we act upon it or not, we are connecting the energy of the will with the energy of love.

Psychosynthesis theory describes the good will as a synthesis of the archetypes or energies of Love and Will. An act of good will made towards someone is a dynamic and joy-filled process that fosters understanding and co-operation. When we tune into the good will we recognise that whatever we do, it is part of the greater whole of human relations. The good will has been described as "love in action". In terms of human relations, so long as we only do to others what we would have them do to us, we are tuning into the energy of the good will. The good will, however, is not just being soft and nice, it is dynamic and active.

Imagine what we would be like if we had no good will at all. We would not be able to actively express love, we would take actions that promote our own interests at the expense of others, we might be suspicious and defensive, judgemental, prejudiced, indifferent to the suffering of others, isolated and so on. On the other hand, we could have too much good will. People would walk all over us, or we might be overly helpful to the point of interference, or we might never be able to say no. We would be so nice we would be really sickly. In fact, this isn't really "good will" at all but an example of the will when it has been hijacked, as it were, by a subpersonality.

With just the right amount of good will we create a true balance between both love and will, we are co-operative and helpful and exhibit all the qualities of "right human relations". At each and every moment, all of us have the choice as to whether we want to exhibit good will or not. As always, we have those three options we've previously delineated—yes, no, or not for now. Right now, we can choose which of these options we wish to take. If we choose to say "yes" to the good will, there will naturally be times when we do not succeed. But whenever this happens, we can always choose to come back to it, centring ourselves again and becoming once more infused with the energy of good will.

> After preparation ... Relax and centre yourself. Think of times in your life when you have missed an opportunity or caused pain to yourself or someone else through your lack of will. Picture these events as vividly as possible and allow the associated feelings to affect you ...
>
> Now write down a list of these times in your life with which you have just connected. Let yourself really desire to change yourself so that you have more will ... [write]
>
> Reflect on all the opportunities and benefits there would be both for yourself and others if your will was strengthened. Think clearly what these advantages would be, then write them down. Allow the feelings aroused by these anticipated advantages to really

affect you. Feel the joy that these opportunities could give you, the satisfaction you would feel if you were stronger willed. Let yourself really feel your desire to become stronger in this way ...

Finally picture yourself as having a strong will. Imagine yourself acting in every situation with firm decisions, focused intention and clear awareness. Visualise yourself walking, talking, sitting and simply being in a way that exhibits your mastery over the will. You are strong, yet subtle, firm yet kind, acting with skill and discrimination.

Realise you can use this technique to strengthen your will whenever you choose ... [write]

¶ BREAK

Freedom

There are two kinds of freedom, freedom from and freedom for. These are well illustrated by the examples shown in the accompanying table.

FREEDOM FROM	FREEDOM FOR
conditioning	pursuit of positive goals
the past	the future
external authority	manifestation of positive interests
patterns of reaction	manifesting real preferences
compulsive behaviour	learning to be free
the need to escape	courage
dependency on others	autonomy
involuntary acts	spontaneity
self-denial	self-acceptance

Freedom from allows us to deal with the past, all our conditioning and learning, and make decisions in the present moment, not unconnected to our previous knowledge and learning but not blindly controlled by these factors.

Freedom for allows us to see into the future and connect with our potential, to make decisions in the present moment with a clear insight into how our potential may manifest. We need both freedom from and freedom for.

In a sense, we all take the conditioning that some things are "sinful". This concept of sin is something we need freedom from. The word is derived from a Greek word that meant "missing the mark". In other words, the only true sin is to miss the mark, that is, to deviate from our true, inner function, our purpose or true will.

As we learn to connect more deeply with our inner purpose, we begin to get a sense of our true will as the deepest, most spiritual and yet most manifest sense of our purpose for being incarnated. True will manifests itself in steps that we take towards its unfoldment. It is a distant goal yet each conscious step we tread this path.

The most important use of freedom for is for the manifestation of this true will. The more freedom to choose you acquire, the more you find yourself doing just that, feeling sufficiently free to be able to make positive, life-enhancing choices that manifest your inner purpose and guidance.

> After preparation ... Choose something you really want to do. Whatever you choose, find for yourself which desire is the strongest in you at this present moment. Write this desire at the top of your paper ...
>
> Close your eyes and say the desire over to yourself several times: "I want [whatever it is]." As you say this, allow a symbol or image for this desire to emerge in your consciousness. Don't force it, just let the image appear. And don't censor it, whatever emerges is the right image for you at this moment. Draw a simple representation of your image or symbol, colouring it appropriately if you so desire ...
>
> Close your eyes and imagine you are standing on top of a hill. Stretching before you is a perfectly straight road that slopes down into and crosses a valley, then climbs up a hill that you can see in the distance. At the end of the road, at the top of the distant hill, you can see a large sign that incorporates your symbol ...
>
> Start walking down the road, taking your time but not deviating at all from the straight road that leads through the valley and up the other hill. Be aware of any distractions that occur, whether they be, for example, a beautiful flower that beckons you to stop and look at it or a demonic figure that tries to pull you from the path. Be aware of these distractions but do not follow them. Keep to the

road, walking with determination towards your goal at the top of the far hill ...

As you climb the distant hill, look ahead and see your image, your symbol, getting larger and larger as you get closer to it. Keep walking up the hill until you reach the top, by which time your symbol has assumed gigantic proportions. When you arrive in front of it make a clear affirmation of your desire, for example: "This is my desire to [whatever it is]." Allow the energy of the symbol to infuse through your whole body, to penetrate into your feelings and to fill your thoughts ...

Become the symbol ...

When you are ready, open your eyes and write about your experience. Make a note of the distractions from the path as well as how you felt when you reached your goal ... [write]

This exercise can be performed over and over, either with the same desire symbol or with other wishes and desires as they become uppermost. It helps direct your consciousness towards your desire, and helps your dream come true. And sometimes the symbol can even be transformed along the way.

---------- ¶ BREAK ----------

The helmsman

As previously mentioned, Assagioli liked to use the analogy of the will as being like the helmsman guiding a ship, providing the direction rather than the power for moving the vessel forward. It is certainly powerful analogy and practised it can also be most enjoyable.

> After preparation ... Imagine you are on a sailing ship, out in a vast ocean, with no land visible in any direction. Let yourself be carried by the ship, taking you where it will for a while ...
> Then let your sense of purpose be present for you (even if, at this time, you are not that clear what your purpose is). Just let yourself be filled with the sense of purpose ...
> Then realise that you can be the helmsman on this ship, you can take control of the rudder and steer the ship in whatever direction

seems most appropriate to you, so that you are travelling in a direction that leads you closer to your purpose ...

Take the helm, and be the helmsman. Vividly imagine yourself in this role, and allow yourself to fully enjoy the experience of being in control of your ship ... [write]

¶ BREAK

The source of good will

The act of will can be confusing. It's very easy to imagine that if we show determination or concentration or are able to focus on something, that this is the will itself. It is not. It is very important to distinguish, for instance, one-pointedness from the will; because of the will we might be able to concentrate or be one-pointed or whatever, but those qualities are not the will itself. The will doesn't in any way need those qualities to exist, it exists alone.

As with meditation, we need to be able to concentrate, to attend to our consciousness, to hold ourselves still, to turn off all our inner dialogues, to achieve a state where we become uncluttered with things that draw us away from the silent oneness of ourselves, the silent oneness within. That silent oneness within, the goal of meditation, is the source of the will. When we can reside in that place, when we reach that place, as soon as an impulse arises for us to take any action, then we are coming away from the source of will, into the world.

> Make yourself as silent as possible ... Reflect: What is the source of all my awareness? Reflect on this question for at least ten minutes ... [write]
>
> Connect to all your experience of the will throughout this lesson, and as you do so open to the spirit of good will. Imagine holding all your experiences in the light of good will. Really picture this ...
>
> Open to good will towards yourself ...
>
> Open to good will towards those nearest to you in your life ...
>
> Open to good will towards all sentient beings ...
>
> Staying connected to good will, exhibit this in some clear and practical way towards the next three people you meet, whatever

level of relationship you have with them. Be aware of the quality of these experiences, whatever the result ... [write]

¶ BREAK

Before starting the next lesson

- Pay attention to your will, how it manifests and how it does not manifest in your life. Consider appropriate actions you can take to develop your will in all its aspects.
- Consider what is the next step (or steps) in the development of will in your life.
- Give yourself at least one hour during which time you cannot be interrupted. Spend this time considering your connection and use of your strong, skilful and good will in light of what you've been exploring in this lesson.

LESSON 9

The realms of spirit and shadow: exploring the heights and depths of the psyche

In this lesson we explore how throughout all the highs and lows we experience in life, the "I" is seen as unconditionally inclusive and constant throughout, regardless. The importance of embracing both the spirit and shadow aspects of the self is stressed. Whatever we believe, it is pragmatically true that we cannot have peaks without troughs, and vice versa. A peak experience may, for instance, be a time when you went beyond your normal, everyday self. A typical trough might be a time of losing control, of feeling like it is not you, as it were, in the driver's seat. All these experiences, whether "good" or "bad", have their rightful and equal importance in the development of your psyche.

Connecting with spiritual energies can lead to personal growth and transformation, and psychosynthesis underscores the need to ground or manifest transpersonal energies in the real world, suggesting that spiritual insights should be shared to have true value. The concept of shadow, encompassing the dark aspects of one's personality, is seen to be in a constant interplay with spirit facing, and facing one's fears and repressed potential is essential for personal and spiritual growth.

In essence, this lesson encourages self-reflection, the integration of both positive and negative experiences, and the recognition of the self's unchanging essence amidst life's ups and downs. It underscores the importance of embracing spirituality and grounding its transformative energies in one's life and in our interconnectedness with others.

The notion of spontaneous spiritual experiences is introduced and the need for personal development to safely handle such spiritual emergence/emergency. The various ways to connect with spiritual energies are discussed and, finally, the lesson presents a meditation exercise involving the growth of a seed, symbolising personal development and the journey towards self-awareness.

Review

- Did you reflect on the actions you can take in the development of your will to deepen your connection?
- Did you give yourself at least one uninterrupted hour considering how the will manifests in your life?

Heights and depths

This first exercise looks at your experiences of heights and depths in your life, and the possibility of a relationship between these apparently different experiences.

> After preparation ... Reflect on the course so far—what for you have been the heights and depths of this psychosynthesis course? ... [write]
>
> Expand these reflections to consider your whole life ... consider your journey through life as we have been exploring it during these lessons ... What have been the high spots (and peaks) in your life? ... And what have been the low spots in your life? ...
>
> Can you find a relationship between the heights and depths of your experiences in life so far? Does it feel to you that there is such a relationship? ...
>
> Now reflect: During your life, what has remained constant? ... [write]

¶ BREAK

Embodiment of energies

When an individual feels able and willing to enter the realms of spirit and shadow, this is where they can access true values and feelings, insights and meaningful connections. From the realm of spirit, we gain knowledge and understanding of our potential for future growth. From the realm of shadow, we can release both blocked and suppressed energies from the past. Accepting both realms allows us to be truly—and wholly—ourselves. As well as heights and depths we can experience something that remains constant throughout, an inclusive self that doesn't dualise or polarise but adds purpose to our experience. We can explore, through our own life experiences, the presence of soul in both our sorrows and joys, and how we may hide not only the shameful but also the sublime within us.

> After preparation ... Standing up, spend a few moments loosening up your body ...
>
> Connect to a time in life when you went beyond yourself, when you had a peak experience ... Recall this in as much detail as possible—where were you? Who were you with? What were the circumstances? ...
>
> Feel the energy associated with this peak time in your body, in your feelings, and in your thoughts, right now ...
>
> Allow your body to make a posture or a movement that expresses this time, allowing your mind and body to be fully infused with the energy ...
>
> Without censoring or judging in any way what comes, let an image emerge in your mind that represents this memory of a peak experience ...
>
> Now let go of the image and the memory, disidentify from your feelings about this time. Notice how willing you are to let go of these memories? ...
>
> Draw the image and make notes about your experience ... [write]
>
> Standing up, connect to a time in your life when you felt driven or compelled by something, a time when you lost control. It may be a time to do with blind desire, lust, anger, fear, jealousy, etc. and recall your own experience in as much detail as possible, filling out the details—where were you? Who were you with? What circumstances? ...

Feel the energy of this experience in your body, in your feelings, and in your thoughts, right now ...

Allow your body to take a posture or make a movement that expresses this time, allowing your mind and body to be fully infused with the energy ...

Now, without censoring or judging what comes, let an image emerge in your mind that represents this memory of a dark, driven time in your life ...

Now let go, disidentify from the energy and feelings of this memory ... How willing are you to let go this time? ...

Shake this memory right off! (A vigorous shake!) ...

Draw the image and make notes about your experience ... [write]

We will work more with these images, but for now, take a

———————————— ¶ BREAK ————————————

The images

After preparation ... Put the two images you drew in the last exercise side by side in front of you. Reflect on the following:

How do the images relate (if they relate at all)? ...

Which are you most attracted to? Which has most energy? ...

Which are you most afraid of? Which do you feel most disconnected from? ...

Consider again: Which has more energy? ...

What have you learned from looking at the two drawings together? ... [write]

———————————— ¶ BREAK ————————————

Spiritual energies

There are many ways for us to connect with the transpersonal or spiritual realms of energy. Meditation is an obvious way; other ways include dance, devotion, concentration, loving sex, aesthetic ecstasy, compassion and shock. There are also many techniques and exercises that have been devised to help us connect with the spiritual, and psychosynthesis uses many of these.

As well as connecting with spiritual energies, we can also manifest them in the world. There is little point in us getting into contact with the spiritual unless we are going to utilise its transforming qualities in ourselves and our world. Psychosynthesis emphasises this need for the grounding or manifestation of transpersonal energies. A spiritual treasure, whatever form it takes, is only truly meaningful when it is "brought back to the world". The rich jewel that an explorer finds is of no value unless he brings it home and shares its splendour with others.

Of course, sometimes just connecting with the transpersonal realms can be enough. We might, for example, feel low and purposeless in our lives, then through a spiritual connection we might find there is hope and meaning after all. Or it might just be to know something more than mundane reality exists is enough. But even if the spiritual connections we make only transform something inside us, it is nevertheless true that these energies will bring into manifestation better human relations. It is inevitable that if we, as individuals, transform ourselves in some way, that transformation will affect those with whom we come into contact.

When we connect with and manifest the transpersonal, we are potentially more able to do our "true will", to make our lives more purposeful. The "higher" or "deeper" Self that is in touch with the Universal Self becomes more manifest through us, so we are truly co-operating with evolution. Then our own psychosynthesis can more readily happen, for we are aligned with rather than fighting against this natural current. And, in a truly dynamic sense, we find our everyday lives are improved. We feel more whole, more meaningful, happier, and those around us can share in our good fortune.

Sometimes the emergence of transpersonal or spiritual energies is not chosen or allowed in some active way, however. The energies "burst in upon us", as it were, in a totally spontaneous way. It has already been made clear that one of the aims of psychosynthesis is to help us to make more connection with the transpersonal. Another aim is to help us deal with the results of more spontaneous emergence of spiritual energies, sometimes called spiritual emergence/emergency.

When energy comes upon us unexpectedly, it can be a very positive experience. We may experience transformative "highs" or quite simply feel a silent "grace" pervading our lives. Sometimes, however, when such energies emerge unexpectedly, it is as if they are too much for the personality to cope with and we are "blown out". If we are fairly well-prepared, we can withstand these blowouts and find ways of utilising the energy. If we are not prepared, then such energies can lead to all sorts of strange distortions of attitude and behaviour. We might think we are literally "god", we might believe we are chosen in some way; we might become inflated in our sense of self. In extreme cases, this can even lead to dangerous behaviour both to ourselves and to others. Many murderers say they have been "spoken to" in some way. Perhaps in some cases the initial contact was genuine enough, but the personality was not able to cope with the energy and consequently it was channelled into a distorted message. Because of this danger, even if only manifested in a mild and fairly harmless way, as is usually the case, psychosynthesis emphasises work on the personality.

If you recognise the danger of any such happening, if you haven't already done so, this would be a good time to find a psychosynthesis or other suitably equipped therapist. No one should have to go through such difficult times without appropriate help and support. The clearer we become in our personalities, the more able we are to deal with and constructively utilise our emerging transpersonal energies, whether chosen or spontaneous.

> After preparation ... Reflect on what you have just read.
>
> Consider: Which methods and techniques do you know work best for you personally to connect to transpersonal or spiritual realms? ...
>
> In what ways do you align with, and in what ways do you fight the processes of nature? ...
>
> What are the benefits to you in contacting transpersonal or spiritual realms? ... [write]

--- ¶ BREAK ---

Grounding energy

The following exercise is a great way of anchoring your energy to the core of the earth.

> After preparation ... Sit upright, let the base of your spine become really heavy, and see it as an anchor. Imagine the anchor goes down into the earth, attached by a light but strong cord to your whole body. Let it pass in its own way through layers of rock and sediment

and anything else it comes to until it finally reaches the core of the earth, then hook it in there. Let it find its own way down and hook to the centre in a natural way, don't force it …

Feel yourself hooked into the planet's core, the planet's energy of which you are a part …

You can extend this exercise by having your feet flat on the ground, and imagining that they have openings on the bottom. Draw energy up through them as you inhale, circulate this energy through your body, then as you exhale let it go back down into the earth. Then you are circulating earth energy through your body. Cycling and recycling this energy will really connect you to the earth …

We are all, individually, a bit like "growths" on the earth's surface, little "blips" sticking out, like hairs on the globe-shaped body of our mother planet. Each "hair" or "blip" is as important as any other and each hair has the potential to grow to its fullest height. You can let this happen through you.

¶ BREAK

Being at peace

This is an easy mindfulness exercise that grounds you internally and connects you to the self behind all identifications. It is a simplified disidentification practice, not to replace the practice you've already been performing but as an alternative approach that can easily be shared with others.

Pay attention to the rhythmic flow of your breathing without trying to change it or force it in any way. Just let yourself freely and easily breathe for a while …

Say to yourself: "My body is at peace." Be aware of any sensations in your body but do not try to suppress them in any way …

Next affirm silently to yourself: "My emotions and feelings are at peace." Do not suppress any emotions that arise, simply be aware of them and let them pass …

Then silently affirm: "My thoughts are at peace." Notice whatever thoughts arise but do not become attached to them …

Visualise yourself as perfectly silent. Be at peace in a perfectly silent, peaceful world …

Silently affirm: "I have sensations, emotions, feelings, thoughts, but I, as an individual Soul, am eternally at peace and at one with the universal rhythm" …

Realise the truth of this statement.

Qualities of the self

Once we realise the great benefits to our world and ourselves when we contact the transpersonal realms, we want to know how we can do it more often and more effectively. As has been said, there are many ways of achieving such a connection, and we use many of these when it is suitable to the unfoldment of any individual's psychosynthesis. It is best to find ways that are appropriate for you—"different strokes for different folks" (or "different scenes for different genes"). In an earlier lesson, you learned how important self-identification is, and the exercise offered a good way of disidentifying from the personality and identifying with the self. This technique is one of the most effective ways of connecting with the spiritual.

In the first instance, by dis-attaching in this way, we are bringing ourselves to our centre, which in itself opens us up to such energy. Then we are also "calling in" or "invoking" the self, our distinct and unique "I". When we move closer to becoming "a centre of pure self-awareness and of will" then we are moving more into the spiritual realms and are thus more able to channel this energy into our personality and, through us, into our world. When we are the self, we are aligned with the Self and are thus making the ultimate individual connection to Spirit itself.

It is important to distinguish the Self from the superconscious. The superconscious is a section of the whole unconscious and is, in fact, an artificial division. Our experience tells us that in reality the unconscious is not divided into sections. But for convenience it is most useful to make the three distinctions, as is done in the psychosynthesis map. The superconscious (or "higher unconscious") is a description for that part of the unconscious that contains energies of a higher frequency than those of the contents of the lower unconscious. This is not saying that one is better than the other, but merely making a distinction to aid understanding.

The Self, on the other hand, is the central reality of a being, the innermost centre where they are completely individual and at the same time connected to everyone and everything else. The "self" (with a small "s") is, as it were, an outpost of the Self (with a capital "S"). The experience of this spiritual Self gives a sense of freedom and expansion to the individual, bringing connection, revelation and spiritual maturity.

The Self never changes in essence; it is "that which remains when all else is gone". The superconscious is constantly changing, however, both as the Self radiates energy into it and then, in turn, it radiates energy into the personality. If we say the Self is like the sun, then the superconscious is the sun's rays, flowing to earth and giving life. We may each have our own individual experience of the sun, but, in reality, it is one sun that illuminates us all.

The Self is constantly radiating qualities into the superconscious. These "soul qualities" include: Love, Truth, Beauty, Joy, Courage, Trust, Ecstasy, Delight, Unity, Calm, Compassion, Peace, Loyalty, Freedom, Risk, Power, Simplicity, Vitality, Understanding, Humour, Patience, Service, Wonder, Eternity, Vitality and so on.

In the superconscious, all these qualities remain in their "pure form", undistorted in any way. As they come through to the middle unconscious and the personality, they become distorted. When we talk about the "distortion" of qualities, we do not mean they go wrong or are bad in any way. It is simply that, in our usual personality state we do not either experience or express these qualities in a clear way. How often have you given or received totally unadulterated, pure Love or Trust? We might be close to the pure experience, but there will still be something else operating at the same time. If a quality becomes even more "distorted" it can take on a "negative" form. Love can become possessiveness, or jealousy, for example, or Trust might become jealousy or slavery.

At first sight, we might think that the distortion of qualities in this way is a very negative experience. On the contrary, however, psychosynthesis teaches us that it is, in fact, very positive. If we can face our possessiveness, for instance, and deal with it appropriately, then it can transform into its underlying quality, or at the very least, some of the transforming energies of that quality will be made manifest.

¶ BREAK

Motivation and intention

If we attempt to manifest any transpersonal energy or quality into the world, it is ineffective so long as it is not grounded through the personality. Nothing can happen without a connection to ground. We have to clearly connect with our transpersonal energies and find ways to effectively bring them into the world. However bright or illuminating our insights and realisation might be, if the light is not radiated then it cannot help light our path, let alone anyone else's.

When we understand the difference between motivation and intention, we can learn to ground our energies much more effectively. Intention essentially comes from a connection to the Self. Motivations, on the other hand, come from our reactions to the outside world, and are "chosen" by subpersonalities. Motivation and intention can actually be the same thing, or at very least be closely connected, but very often they are not.

Motivations are usually exclusive and are what push us into partial, un-centred and often ill-considered decisions and actions. They are a reaction, and often a victim kind of reaction at that. Intentions, on the other hand, are more about getting our deeper needs fulfilled. These needs are not so exclusive and are more about manifesting the Self and our true will or purpose. If I am motivated to want a banana then nothing else will do. I will get angry or upset if I don't get it. If I can contact my inner need more clearly, I might find it is actually for fruit. I can now happily eat an orange and fulfil my purpose.

Whether we are dealing with the deepest intention of the Self or a simple desire or motivation from a subpersonality, we need a definite plan to fulfil it. This plan will tell us how we can go about manifesting or grounding our desire. This plan might include a need for us to be strong willed or we might just have to let go and accept what is. We might need to be single-minded, or we might need to deal with some emotional state before it can happen. Once we have done the preparatory work, we are then able to ground our transpersonal energies.

There are several easy ways to ground energy, many of which you have already met in previous lessons:

- simply expressing the experience;
- writing, and/or drawing;
- evening reviews (going over the past day and looking how you performed, not as a judgemental exercise but in order that you might

function more effectively through knowledge of how you habitually perform);
- meditation, either on the object of the will itself or a symbol you have constructed to represent the will;
- evocative word cards, sometimes called "self-advertising"—you write your desire (in words or symbols) on postcards and stick them up around your home in places where you will frequently see them—just as with commercial advertising, constant exposure has an effect on the unconscious;
- free or automatic drawing;
- creating a mantra and constantly chanting or repeating it to yourself;
- specific acts in your life, for example going to beautiful places;
- finding an object to represent what happened.

The aim of grounding is, ultimately, to co-operate with our personal and transpersonal evolution. We can help in that process by taking responsibility for the creation of our life, using our abilities to fulfil our real inner needs, and to ground our inspirations and insights. The most effective ways of grounding energy come from your own life situations. If you have never gone fishing there's little point (in the short term anyway) of grounding a need for fish through fishing. You'd do better to fit the need into your life situation and experience, that is, go to the local fishmonger!

> Consider this section in light of what you learned so far about the will. Reflect on the relevance to grounding of the process of willing. How do you best ground your choices for your life? [write]

---¶ BREAK---

A bag of shadow

The American philosopher Robert Bly offers us a down-to-earth analogy for understanding our shadow. He makes the comparison with a bag that we haul round with us throughout our life. This shadow bag is filled with everything we have repressed, everything we don't like about ourselves and push into the background, every memory forgotten, and all our instincts and desires that are too hot to handle. We carry this bag on our shoulders, continuously adding more as we go through life. It is only through conscious psychological work on oneself that an individual can start to remove some items from this bag. To empty it could be described as a lifetime's work, and the chances of ever completely emptying it are extremely slim if not impossible.

The *Oxford English Dictionary* gives many different meanings to the word shadow. The meaning we are particularly interested in here is shadow in a psychological sense. This is described as the dark aspect of personality formed by those fears and unpleasant emotions which, being rejected by the ego and subpersonalities of which an individual is conscious, exist in the lower unconscious. Some of the other definitions the OED gives for the word shadow are worth reflecting on. Read the following definitions and write about what shadow means to you in your own life:

- The darkness of night; the growing darkness after sunset.
- The image cast by a body intercepting light.
- What is fleeting or ephemeral.
- An unreal appearance; a delusive semblance or image; a vain and unsubstantial object of pursuit. Often contrasted with substance.
- Something of opposite character that necessarily accompanies or follows something else, as shadow does light.
- One that constantly accompanies or follows another like a shadow. A companion whom a guest brings without invitation.

The psychosynthesis view of the shadow emphasises that all the materials that we repress are useful to us, are the things in our life that make us who we are, individuals on a journey of soul-making. We also find it very useful to see our shadow has different aspects or levels, depending upon what it "shadows".

---¶ BREAK---

Layers of shadow

The psychosynthesis egg diagram (see p. 33) shows the human psyche split into three distinct areas, drawn in such a way that the dividing lines appear to convey the notion of levels. Also, as you have learned, all areas of the unconscious have equal importance. Remember that the lower unconscious represents psychic material that has become what psychologists usually understand by shadow. Psychosynthesis suggests a much more complex shadow than that, and the egg diagram can help us understand the different levels of shadow. The "regular shadow", as already described, comprises material from the individual's past, the dark aspect of personality formed by those fears and unpleasant emotions which, being rejected by the self or persona of which an individual is conscious and which exist in the middle unconscious.

The shadow aspect of the higher unconscious involves a process that in psychosynthesis is called "the repression of the sublime". The idea is that we put our potential into shadow as much as our traumas. Because we fear being who we really are, expressing our full potential, we divert and repress these energies. But, of course, we cannot just wish fears away, but to make our fears more conscious is a useful task to approach with the spirit of inquiry.

For instance, if we are going to be truly ourselves it entails a certain responsibility, a heavy-duty responsibility that we may naturally and understandably fear. Such responsibility can be too much and we shy away from it, or we build a false structure around ourselves. One of our biggest fears is the fear of death, yet in one sense we truly die each day many times over, as we change and grow and become different. Even in a physical sense we have many millions of cells dying within us each day. In around seven years from now new cells will have replaced every single cell in your entire body. Apparently, all the cells in your eyes are continuously renewed within a few days. Yet psychosynthesis suggests that there is something that remains, something beyond the contents of the body and personality. To live with this belief offers us the opportunity to embrace each day anew.

It is also possible to fear losing our individuality, particularly from the ego's perspective. Surrendering to the universal can sound terrifying. Of course, if it were possible to lose your soul that would be a calamity, but to lose your separateness and false boundaries can be a blessing. It may seem paradoxical when psychosynthesis is constantly stressing the importance of individuality and being oneself to say you have to lose your individuality, but, when you truly connect this paradox appears quite sane.

If we resist our inner strength and power, we are not making a real distinction between personal and soul power. Personal power comes and goes, but soul power remains (whether we lose our awareness of it or not). If it is always there, is it not better to utilise it than fear it? But what if you misuse your power? You might end up hurting others. You may fear intruding on another person's process in an inappropriate way, even harmfully. You need to recognise you are a soul, you are the source in your universe. The process of life can be trusted through inclusion, centring and synthesis.

Of course, all this is a tall order—we are talking a lifetime of commitment to one's process, not a quick-fix therapy. This is a lot to ask: you may not, in your personality, feel adequate, or deserving, or "good enough", but your purpose, once you have connected to it, will not be removed or balked at. The best course of action is to stop looking for results, just follow your unfolding life a step at a time, and you will find all the energy you need. You can imagine that you have to be perfect before you can serve, indeed, before you can be truly yourself. Yet perfection is just being who you are; all the so-called "good" aspects and "bad" aspects are all perfect for you at this moment. Allow and trust a lot more in yourself as you are.

The most insidious fear of all is the fear of success, of being who you really are. Various ways are suggested so that an individual or group can work on this by developing will, through disidentification, and actively working on the expression of purpose in a calmer, more centred way. This allows soul energies to manifest more effectively, instead of being diverted and distracted. Ultimately, fear is our worthiest opponent, offering us unequalled opportunities for growth.

The middle unconscious includes how shadow controls you now. For instance, many of our behaviour patterns are controlled by unmet needs that have been repressed into the higher or lower unconscious and now exert their powerful and controlling influence. It is these repressed needs that are behind the building of character, the personal history as seen through the body and personality of an individual. Reich's notion of character armour fits here well for just as the body is rigidified and distorted through the creation of physical armouring against emotional as well as physical pain, so the psychosynthesis egg is said to rigidify and become more or less porous. In one sense, the dotted boundary shown on the psychosynthesis egg diagram is the body itself.

The Self is put at both top and bottom of egg, and for that matter anywhere else on the edge of the egg, including around the middle unconscious with as much validity as anywhere else. The implications of this are apparent, that all the areas of the egg are the work of the Self. In other words, the shadow is a creation of the Self. This ties in well with the paradoxical idea, held by many religious systems from the ancient Taoists onwards, that the difficulties and problems we experience in life are in fact opportunities. At the very least they offer the possibility of working on the issue to build strength, grow and even become more effective and integrated in life.

All three realms or areas of the psychosynthesis egg are equally of spirit and of shadow. The inclusive psychosynthesis model is very different from dualistic models of the realms of spirit and shadow as it takes a "both/and" rather than an "either/or" stance. It does this precisely by including both spirit and shadow into a larger container (a "synthesis"), which by definition is more than the sum of its contents.

> Reflect on your relationship with the different aspects of spirit and shadow within yourself ...

---------------- ¶ BREAK ----------------

The ritual dance of spirit and shadow

Ritual dance is one of the oldest forms of dance and, somewhat paradoxically, may not include anything we might usually call dance. Picture one of our ancestors realising that not only are they moving, but more—that they can move in any direction and form. They realise that moving with choice allows them to create realities beyond the mundane and to invoke forces that aid life—whether in childbirth, lighting fires, finding food or whatever. This "awakened" person has become a magician or shaman. Then, because they are successful in fulfilling their basic survival needs, they can dance for healing, choosing to become a healer, or simply for their own or for someone else's pleasure. A performer, an artist is born.

Every time we choose to move or dance and focus our attention on the moving or dancing itself, we have the opportunity to by-pass our everyday states of consciousness. Our habitual inner dialogue of unfocused chatter and emotional reaction may be turned off (or at least turned down!). No longer controlled by our conscious minds, we may more readily enter realms of value and feeling.

When we dance in this way, we are using our abilities to focus and move to enter altered states of consciousness in which we co-operate with rather than resist the unfoldment of our inner processes. These inner processes, rooted in the unconscious, give us access to the two interconnected realms of spirit and of shadow. Dancing through the realm of the shadow, we release energies, blocked or suppressed, from our past, then use these energies to clear our current consciousness. Dancing through the realm of spirit, we gain knowledge and understanding of our potential—in other words, we can divine our future possibilities.

The two realms of spirit and shadow are the territories of all shamanic or magical dancing. Entering these realms, we connect with our constantly evolving inner world, moving and changing as the body decodes the messages and signals from the unconscious. We may start to feel whole (and healed) through quite simply being ourselves.

How easy it is to miss the relevance of ritual when we see it as something obscure, strange or even frightening. We all perform rituals every day in our lives, from the rituals of rising in the morning through to the ritual of going to bed at night. If we make our rituals conscious then we empower ourselves. We give ourselves the opportunity to change and restructure our daily life rituals so they serve rather than hinder us.

We can create and perform rituals that help us connect with our potential and release our blocked energies. These rituals do not have to be complicated: for example, you could create a ritual by choosing to dance to discover the meaning of a dream, with no preconceptions, simply allowing the movement to flow from an image in the dream.

To create ritual dances is nothing special, they do not require the learning of any particular dance or life skills, and are for everyone. All you have to do is choose to bring consciousness into your movement. It's not even that you have got to think of yourself as a dancer, and this sort of practice is open to you even if you are certain that you are a non-dancer in the traditional sense. This is something even those of you who may have always insisted that you can't dance can still do!

Start with the dance of life: spend a day looking at how you perform the everyday rituals of your life. Are these rituals done with consciousness and joy; are you performing them in a way you choose? Is there anything that stops you from choosing this? Both the ability to choose (spirit) and what stops you from remaining conscious and choosing (shadow) are the substance of ritual dance. Bring your awareness onto both and allow the dance of your "body-self" to flow through you. It may be a transforming experience.

> After preparation ... Create a ritual that exemplifies and furthers your relationship with both the realm of spirit and that of shadow. (If you really, really don't like dancing, make up your own version of this involving at least some kind of movement.) ... [write]

--- ¶ BREAK ---

Inner ecology

Human ecology is about the interaction of people with each other and with their environment, including all our interconnectedness and all our interpenetrability. That's all inside us as well as outside us. What a lot to carry. So we get caught up, through our subpersonalities, in emotional dramas, irrational mental fantasies and soul-less interactions. We experience a triple separation:

- separated within ourselves (with all the attendant inner dialogue this creates, oh 'good' me oh 'bad' me!);
- separated from ourselves (with large parts of us lost in shadow);
- and separated from the Self within us (so disconnected from our highest and deepest aspirations).

Or so it seems at those times, but nothing can truly be in opposition to the unfolding universe, however it may temporally appear.

What if we move away from a dualistic worldview and take a more unifying, psychosynthesis perspective by considering that everything is just as it is, each person and event perfect in itself? From that viewpoint, we don't have to put some idea of "destiny", "fate", or even "god" into it to say that things are meant to be; it's simply that things unfold as they unfold. And, of course, if there is no "god" directing everything then it is highly likely there is no opposite force trying to spoil things either.

From this perspective, the point of psychosynthesis isn't to make the world different, rather it is to make us aware of how the world is so that we have increased choice about how we interact with it. If we can do anything about the state of the world, it is to come to that place of acceptance where what is, simply is. The aim of such a perspective is not to make us into passive observers, or disempower us, but to offer insight and connections that enable us to make clearer choices. At a deep level this means to realise the personal and Spiritual (or "Transpersonal") Will are not separate within or without us.

If we look further from this inclusive, unified position (rather than a dualistic one) it offers us an insight into the dynamic of synthesis. Rather than the opposing poles remaining separate and the best that can happen is to find a place somewhere between the two, somewhere that is neither one or the other (an "either/or" state), from a synthesising perspective we move to a different position where we include both poles in the apparent opposition (a "both/and" state). If, for instance, our thoughts and feelings are in opposition, then we look for a way to bring these two forces together (perhaps through finding ways of activating a stronger connection to a deeper intent) rather than holding them apart and trying to find some (imagined) middle ground.

If we set something against something else from the viewpoint of the personality there is separation and conflict, but this is an opportunity for growth, particularly as the perceived separation highlights the conditions at play and offers us clearer perspective on the choices available. Separation then enables us to have some clearer choices about how we view ourselves in the world, and our understanding of ourselves and, most importantly gives us the opportunity to come back to ourselves. In words from the Western Mystery Tradition: we are separated for the sake of love and the chance of union.

Human ecology is about interaction, interconnectedness and interpenetrability. Truth is, if we inquire deeply, we find that ecological responsibility is not "out there" but within ourselves. If we are, at a fundamental level, all one (or at the very least "all on this journey together") then we each have to take individual responsibility for what we project into the world, what we prefer to see as remote and not to do with us, not "our fault". Embracing what apparently separates us gives us a great opportunity to take this responsibility and make our choices life-affirming, moving us towards rather than away from the unity of Self that underpins all, the essential connection for a true and deep ecological awareness.

One flower among many

After preparation ... Paying particularly attention to being as relaxed and centred as possible ... get an image of a seed, seeing it in a dark, muddy environment, beneath a pool, embedded and waiting to grow ...

Identify with the seed, become it, feel the dark, wet, silent environment you inhabit ... As you do this, become aware also of your urge to grow, to fulfil yourself ... Start to experience your growth, your roots pushing blindly down into the mud for nourishment and anchorage, and your growing tip pushing up through the mud ...

Experience now breaking through mud not into air but into water. Be aware you have completed a first stage of growth, but still have far to travel ... Take some time to consolidate your roots, knowing their vital importance for your future growth ...

Now continue your journey as a growing seed: as your roots grow deeper, your growth proceeds upwards, sometimes strongly, sometimes not, but continuously, through the water until you reach the surface, the clean air and the light ...

Experience yourself growing leaves on the surface while drawing on the dark fertile sustenance of your roots ...

Be aware of yourself forming buds in the air, then the warmth of the sun shining down, gently opening your buds ...

Become a flower, opening in the bright sunlight ...

Then realise you are one flower among others. Look around you at the other beautiful flowers, also blossoming above the water ... Spend some little time with this image and the feelings it evokes ...

Start to let go of the image but stay in touch with what you are experiencing now ... Be aware it is only an image and be willing to let the image drop away while you stay in touch with what you are experiencing ...

Know that you are this image and you are more than this ... Don't try to work it out, be with yourself in this experience. Experience the Self that is not the image ...

Who is aware right now? Stay with this experience for some time before continuing ... [write]

---- ¶ BREAK ----

Before starting the last lesson

Spend some time (how much is up to you) reading through and considering the material you have covered in the previous lessons. Pay particular attention to your practical and experiential understanding of the concepts presented, including:

- the psychosynthesis egg diagram;
- the journey of life from a psychosynthesis perspective;
- the psychosynthesis body, feelings, mind model;
- subpersonalities and the inner child;
- identification and disidentification;
- the process of willing;
- polarities of light and shadow.

As you review this work, make notes of anything you feel unclear or uncertain about, and also note anything that has particular significance or meaning for you in your life journey ... [write]

---- ¶ BREAK ----

The course so far

Reflect on your body, feelings and thoughts as they have been engaged during this course. How are they engaged now, at this moment? ...

Considering the journey that you have undertaken to study and practise psychosynthesis, and particularly this course, ask yourself: What old patterns did I repeat during this time? What new ways did I try out? ... [write]

Reflect on the range of emotions you have been feeling ... delight, sadness, anger, boredom, excitement, etc. ... now let go of these feelings ...

What insights have you had? ... What has been the meaning for you of the experiences you have had during exercises? ... now let go of these thoughts ...

Consider to what extent your relationship to this course has been just as it has needed to be, including any desires for it to have been different ... to what extent do you accept it as it is? ...

Give yourself at least one uninterrupted hour considering how much you do or do not accept your life as it is.

LESSON 10

Acceptance and change: global issues and embodying leadership

This final lesson stresses the importance of acceptance. The choice between active acceptance rather than passive resignation is emphasised. Reactive responses are compared to having one's strings pulled, while responses rooted in acceptance engage one's deepest values and feelings. From a place of acceptance in the present moment, psychosynthesis supports a personal and interpersonal spirituality that centres on the journey of life, rather than specific goals.

The lesson delves into the concept of ageing, suggesting that becoming an elder is not solely defined by age but by how well one integrates life's lessons. A mature acceptance of oneself and others is seen as a hallmark of wisdom. The inevitability of death is discussed as another major point of separation that an individual must learn to accept. A "facing death meditation" is introduced, encouraging contemplation of mortality as a powerful tool for embracing the present moment.

Self-knowledge is emphasised as emerging from direct experience rather than blind faith. That we are all divine beings is emphasised, and through experiencing this divinity directly you connect to and can express more clearly your unique purpose or "true will", aligning yourself with Universal Spirit.

The concept of personal leadership is introduced, especially the role of leaders in helping others find their true nature rather than trying to direct or control them. Every individual plays a vital role in life, and embracing one's unique role contributes to collective consciousness and human growth. In the context of leadership and global awareness, it is strongly asserted that each and every individual definitely matters and has the power to influence the world positively. The importance of embracing one's role in various individual situations, and one's roles in the community of humankind as well as local communities, are highlighted.

The lesson concludes with a meditation on world healing and the importance of finding the true silence behind and beyond all inner and outer activity.

Review

- Did you reflect on and write on the course so far and what has worked or not for you?
- Did you give yourself at least one uninterrupted hour considering the extent of your acceptance as it is?

Set and setting

For any change to occur you need to recognise what state you are in, and what state your surroundings are in. Sometimes called set and setting, this is simply where we are and whom we are with. If we do not recognise these things, then nothing can change. If we do recognise the circumstances we are in (which is not necessarily as easy as it first may appear), then we have the choice to accept these conditions or not. This isn't resignation but active acceptance. If it is not active acceptance, we can be pretty sure our response is reactive in some way. When we react to something or someone, we are understandably not in control of our lives. A response to something, on the other hand, engages the energy of acceptance and is experienced through our deepest values and most precious feelings.

Psychosynthesis supports a personal and interpersonal spirituality that is more about the journey of life than any particular goals or expectations.

Reflect: What do I accept in my life, and what would I like to change? ... [write]

---¶ BREAK---

Ongoing acceptance

Accepting things does not mean becoming a passive victim, but more actively engaging in the process of what is emerging. Acceptance of this kind, which involves choice, has a relevance to the individual, whether alone, in relationship with others, or while interacting with the world.

Our primary wounding, as we explored earlier, involved our separation from mother, and has been described as the original separation. Interestingly, many creation myths put a separation right at the beginning of the story. Whether this is relevant to an individual or not is a debatable point, but one thing is certain: in being born, we all separated from mother. This experience is at the root of all our anxieties about being at-one with someone or something and our experiencing separation from someone or something. As you have learned, to be at one or to be separated is the basic polarity at the root of subpersonality formation.

The other main time of separation is at the moment of death. That we are all going to die is the other major issue that we have to learn, through our lives, to accept. In a sense we are prepared by the death of others, particularly loved ones, but only an active, inner chosen acceptance allows us to live our lives with the certain knowledge of our own death.

Shakespeare, in his play *Measure for Measure* sums up the psychosynthesis attitude very well when one of the characters says that if they must die, they will encounter darkness as "a bride and hug it in my arms". Another way of expressing this, from the shamanic teachings of Carlos Castañeda, is the idea of using death as an advisor. Certainly, to live life with the ever-present acknowledgement of death can sharpen our experiences.

Reflect on how much has happened during the few minutes you have been reading this. ... [write]

In one sense, probably not a lot happens during a few minutes, particularly if we focus on our individual experience. Much could happen in a few minutes, however: you could die, for instance, or become ill, and so on, but the chances are that these things probably won't happen while you are sitting reading. If we expand our consciousness, however, to include more than just our own individual circumstances, then the answer to what has happened during the few minutes you have been reading this is considerably more profound. For instance, we have travelled many millions of miles in space; a large number of babies have been born; a number of people died (maybe twenty every minute); and so on. These are examples of things we cannot change whether we like it or not. All we can do is accept what is.

Another thing we have to accept is that we are always in the present moment. We only can ever experience the present. I can remember the past (here and now) but I can no longer experience it. I can imagine and predict the future, but (until it happens) I can only experience my fantasies about the future in the present moment. So being always present is something else we cannot change—all we can do is accept what is. That we are always here and now (here being associated with our position in space, and now to our moment in time) is an important experience on the journey towards enlightenment. Indeed, for many mystical approaches, it is not just an experience on the journey, it is the goal itself. So acceptance plays an important part in our transpersonal development as well as our personal growth.

> Reflect on this moment, now... don't do anything with your experience; whatever you are thinking, feeling, sensing, whatever you are experiencing, just reflect on being here and now in this moment ...
>
> Now reflect on this moment ... And this moment ... and this ...
>
> Reflect now on the time that apparently passes from one moment (this moment) until the next. You might like to use a clock or watch to time five minutes, and simply watch your experiences through this time ...
>
> Now ask yourself: what remains the same? ... [write]

What remains the same is not the content of our perception, whether that's sensations, feelings or thoughts. What remains the same is not what we focus on, nor how we focus. What remains the same is the source of our attention, the source of all we perceive. Yet, paradoxically, we cannot find a place or space within us that is this source, nor can we fix it in time.

--- ¶ BREAK ---

A question of ageing

We can now explore the last two turns of the wheel on the journey of life, the one from mature adult to elder, and the final one from elder into death. Of course, not everyone (either developmentally or literally!) reaches the status of "elder", but with certainty everyone reaches death.

One of the major features of a life that can confer the status of elder on someone is not what age they reach (although they may well deserve the title then just for having reached a certain age) but how well they have integrated the lessons of life. This is not to say anyone is better or worse than another, just that we all live unique and idiosyncratic lives, developing more in some areas and less in others. Perhaps the truest sign of integration and the wisdom that comes with it is recognising that we are just right as we are, wherever and however we have developed through life. Certainly, many old people exhibit great acceptance of themselves and others.

> Reflect on wisdom ...
> In your experience, what makes a person wise? ... [write]

--- ¶ BREAK ---

The ageing process

You will need a mirror for the following exercise, preferably one you can easily hold.

> Reflect: How old are you? ... how old do you feel? ...
> How old did you feel ten years ago: older, younger or the same as now? ... How old did you feel when you were in your late teens? ... [write]

> Reflect back on your childhood: what was your skin like? how did it feel to touch your skin? … Feel your own skin now—touch your hands, face, any other exposed areas of your skin—how is it different from when you were a child? What feelings, or other responses and reactions do you have to doing to this? … [write]
>
> Imagine you are the child you were, standing before a mirror … see your hair, eyes, face in your imagination …
>
> Now look in a mirror—look at yourself now—look at your hair, your eyes and your face—what difference has ageing made to your appearance? …
>
> What difference is there in your own response to your appearance, now as compared to then? How do you feel about your appearance now? … [write]
>
> Consider your whole body now … how has it changed since you were younger? What changes has your body gone through? …
>
> What changes have there been in your feelings about life, and feelings about yourself? What changes have there been in your ideas about life, and ideas about yourself? … [write]
>
> What about your ideas about ageing? What has changed in your responses to ageing since you were younger? …
>
> How do you feel, now you are ageing and know it? … [write]

———————— ¶ BREAK ————————

Facing death meditation

Death is always with us. Maybe death is waiting just behind your left shoulder, waiting to tap you—when it does and you look round, you are facing your death. Or, another way of understanding it, death is always just half a breath away, and you could die before you take your next in- or out-breath.

Ensure that you have plenty of time before undertaking the next exercise, and read it through a couple of times to familiarise yourself with what you are being asked to do. Before starting, consider how you feel about this exercise after reading it through, but before actually doing it.

> Create a circle around yourself, really taking time to imagine and visualise this circle around you … Stand at the centre of this circle

and loosen up, stretch, bounce, do whatever connects you to being physically present in this place right now ...

Step to the edge of your circle and start to and walk round the circumference (in a clockwise direction). Keep walking throughout this meditation ...

As you walk, consider people in your life who have died ... simply reflect on these people and notice how this makes you feel in your body ... what emotions come up? what associated thoughts? ... allow them to be present now ...

Consider times in your own life when you have faced your own death ... illnesses, accidents, depressions ... allow yourself to be aware of associated sensations, feelings and thoughts without indulging in them ...

Still walking around the circle, imagine you are on your own death bed: reflect now on the different ways you can die—peacefully, of old age, in a road accident, younger than expected, with cancer, Aids, from heart failure, from gradual decay, with others, alone in a flat with no one knowing, surrounded by your family, alone in hospital, in an aeroplane, at sea ...

Still walking the circle, consider now, if you had just died, how your corpse might be: reflect on your corpse, lifeless and bloodless ... the skeleton, the bones of your corpse ... the flesh, eaten by worms and insects ... a corpse that has been beaten and hacked into pieces ... a bloody corpse ... a bloated corpse, full of water ... a rotting, smelly corpse, a burnt corpse, consumed with flames ...

Still walking round your circle, now consider the earth ... consider silence ... consider death ... Take as long over this stage as is appropriate to you and your current situation ...

Stop walking now and face into the circle around which you have been walking ... project all of your thoughts, fantasies, feelings, reactions, sensations and responses to death into your circle ...

From where you are now, taking your time to sense and feel this journey as you experience it if you feel OK to do so, walk into the circle, the territory of death and feel its presence ...

Once inside your circle, begin to develop a relationship with death ... locate in your body your contact point with death; where inside you are your responses to death? ... Give yourself over to this experience and express this now as much as you are willing ...

When you are ready, find a gesture, movement or dance that communicates the essence of your relationship with death ...

Dance now your last dance, your dance with death (staying within your circle) ...

When you feel complete, return to the circumference of the circle, turn and acknowledge the presence of death ...

Finally, close the circle in whatever way feels right to you, making sure it is not left open in any way ... then make sounds and stomp around to make sure you feel fully present and alive back in your body.

Only later ... [write]

¶ BREAK

A soul letter

It is not absolutely necessary for this exercise, but if you can get a proper letter-writing pad and envelopes; if not, use a separate sheet of paper, not your usual journal. Write a letter to your soul, expressing whatever comes to you that you'd like to express to soul. Address it as you wish ("Dear Soul ..." for instance) and write it just as if you are writing it to post ... [write]

When it is completed, put it in the envelope, address it (use your imagination!) and then put the letter away somewhere where you will be able to find it later. Don't do anything else with it just now!

¶ BREAK

We are all divine

One of the greatest, and best-known, esoteric maxims is: as above, so below. This statement asserts the essential identity between the creator and the creation. We could say God made man in his own image and Goddess made woman in her own image. This is not really acceptable, however, because it implies a dualism that denies our experience when we connect with our inner world. It would be truer to say Goddess–God made woman–man in its own image, then split this creation into two so that, through this division, the creation may experience love and realise its true essential divine identity.

Self-knowledge has to be a direct experience, not simply a matter of faith. Without denying the importance of faith, it is clear that to have true self-knowledge we must directly experience our own selves. From this experience we may then have a living faith, based on our direct, experienced understanding, which is very different from a blind faith based upon what someone else has told us to be the truth. For some people faith alone might be enough to sustain them and help them develop and grow closer to an understanding of their own inner nature, but if we are to truly know ourselves as one with the divine, we must experience this directly.

Everything we experience can be seen as an opportunity for growth and movement towards self-realisation. Not least among these opportunities are those presented to us through our bodies. The body is a living temple of the soul. It is through our bodies that we incarnate on this planet, and it is only through our bodies that we can interact with the dense matter of existence. It is vital, therefore, that we treat our bodies with all the respect that is due to such a precious temple. Our world is a temple, too, the outer temple in which we experience and express ourselves. We can thus make another connection, that between our inner temple (body) and outer temple (external world). It is as important we treat our outer temple with as much respect as that we give our inner temple. When we abuse our planet, it reflects our abuse of ourselves. When we truly honour our bodies, we inevitably honour our outer temple too.

Whatever we know scientifically, from our planetary perspective we experience the sun as dying each evening and being reborn each morning. If we could stand on the sun, we would realise the light as continuous, at the centre of all activity, including the cycles of the earth. Similarly, from our terrestrial perspective, we experience a similar cycle of life and death. As souls, however, we can realise our continuity, seeing that birth and death are transition points that bring us into and take us out of incarnation on the planet. If we experience this truth, we inevitably see that there is some purpose for coming into incarnation. This purpose is, in essence, to realise our true inner divinity and connection to the deity.

For each of us, as individual souls, however, there is, in any incarnation, a particular purpose for being here. We have special lessons to learn, and until we truly experience and understand our lessons, we continue spiralling through an endless cycle of experiences (and incarnations even), with these lessons being presented to us in numerous different ways. Once a particular lesson is learned, we can then move on to the next lesson. Each step in this unfolding process brings us nearer to the realisation of our purpose or true will, the reason why we are here. For one person the purpose might be to express love in some lofty, abstract sense, for another to express love in caring for sick or handicapped people. Perhaps for someone else it may be to stand against a particular injustice so more truth can be made manifest, for another it might simply be to act as a catalyst for someone else's progress. No individual's purpose is better or worse than another's. The key is to find our own purpose or true will and then to do it. When we achieve this, we have truly aligned ourselves, as souls, with the universal Spirit.

From the "source of all life" right through to the earthliest individual human, it is vital to stress the absolute equality of every manifest being. We are all divine, not in some abstract sense, but in our everyday lives. Whatever we do, we are never disconnected from our essential nature. The myths of gods and goddesses often show us that even divine beings may stray from their purpose and misdirect their energies. We humans are no different! To realise and, more importantly, to manifest our essential divinity, we have to work at it. This is a life-long process and extreme caution is advised when we meet those who would tell us of their great initiations, spiritual attainment, understanding of the true mysteries and so forth. Part of our spiritual development, in finding us our own true nature, is for us to re-own our power from all the masters, secret chiefs, gurus, shamans and the like. Everyone met on the path is at least an equal, and always possibly just the person we need to teach us a particular lesson.

As well as being surrounded by this endless multiplicity of other divine beings masquerading as humans, all other entities in all the universes, whether imagined or real, are truly aspects of the divine. We can always be on the lookout, therefore, for messages, teachings, understanding, not only from other humans or from some direct spiritual inspiration, but also from archangels, angels, demons, animals, plants and rocks! If this sounds fantastic, consider what it means to view the world this way. Whatever we may believe (consciously), our unconscious carries endless possibilities. If we can connect to this realm of the unconscious, we can liberate energies that can enrich our understanding of ourselves and all our potential. We may then realise that everything in our lives is a manifestation from the unconscious. From this viewpoint it is no less strange or fantastic to talk to an archangel than it is to dream of a goldfish.

It is also important with self-development work to remember the sacredness of all life. Everything has its angel, its divine breath, from each individual cell through to the planet earth and the whole universe. Everything is interconnected, nothing in our universe is separate (however temporarily separate it may sometimes appear). To be truly divine ourselves, we cannot deny the divinity of any other being, for to do so would deny our own divinity. We have a collective responsibility to the totality of life. Every time we do anything that is thoughtless, uncaring or off-mark in some way, we lessen the total amount of connection and consciousness on our planet. Conversely, every time we do something with care, whenever we act from our true selves, we add to the pool of positive consciousness on our planet. We are all individually responsible, and each act we take does make a difference. When we live our lives from this true divine perspective, we are working for the collective responsibility, and it is only through realising this collective responsibility that we may start to heal our planet.

Some indigenous peoples recognise soul in their everyday experience. They don't see themselves as separate or superior to nature but recognise the interdependence of all creation and honour this. In this attitude, which is the aspiration of our psychosynthesis work, there is no split between ecology and spirituality. We learn to value nature as dearly as we value our souls.

> Reflect on what makes life sacred for you, and what "takes you away from" or disconnects you from this sacredness. ...
>
> Discover five ways that you can be more connected to both your own and everyone else's divinity. These might be little matters like, for instance, saying thank you more openly and clearly, through to major life issues that you cannot just simply change. Whatever five ways you discover, try to live by these principles very consciously for several days ...
>
> After this time, reflect on how you succeeded with this task, what works and what doesn't work for you ... [write]

¶ BREAK

Wealth

Wealth can be defined as the outcome of changes in the environment that are of benefit to humanity and/or other life forms on an individual or collective basis. By this definition, examples of wealth include a bridge across a river, a chair, a pollution free environment, and so on. They would also include less tangible forms of wealth such as knowledge, understanding, warmth, Joy, and so on, which, despite being non-physical, are nonetheless the most important items of wealth. Money should not be confused with wealth.

Unfortunately, many of our society's concepts and actions are built upon money rather than wealth. With our planet in its current state of crisis, environmentally, socially and politically, it is our clear moral duty as conscious beings to hold as many concepts and to make as many actions as we possibly can to encourage the growth of real wealth, not financial acquisition.

> Reflect on what ways can you help encourage the growth of wealth in your immediate environment ... [write]

¶ BREAK

Care for the soul

Sit on a chair or cushion with a second chair or cushion conveniently placed in front of you, facing in your direction. Imagine that your soul sits on that chair. Without trying too hard, engage your soul in a dialogue. Start by telling it something about what you think, feel or sense ...

When you feel ready, move positions, sit on the chair or cushion opposite and become your soul. Look back at yourself as a personality in the original position, and answer back. Say whatever comes to you ...

At your own pace, allow a dialogue to happen between your personality and your soul. Don't try to make it anything special, or force it in any way, but simply see what happens. And watch for non-verbal messages that might come from the soul chair,

> such as particular body postures, facial expressions, gestures and so on ... [write]

You can use this exercise to bring greater understanding between you and soul, and also to find inner guidance on issues of importance to you. You have to separate the medium from the message. What soul tells you will be the truth, but the way you hear the message can be distorted. Be careful not to expect the advice to be too concrete; it usually isn't, but it should be supportive in at least the long term. It is also important to discriminate, to look for non-verbal reinforcement, any changes in body position or breath patterns that suggest whether the dialogue is working effectively. Also watch for judgements creeping in—the soul is never judgemental towards the personality—firm yes, but angry no.

Try to find ways to express in your daily life what soul tells you so you can check its validity in the real world. Remember you are the soul and you have a personality, not vice versa. Don't worry if the exercise doesn't work too well for you—it certainly does not mean you are without a soul. It might be simply that the exercise is not right for you in some way, or it might be that, at this time in your personal evolution, your soul is choosing to work "undercover" and a dialogue would be inappropriate. Trust that your own process is unfolding as it is meant to and you cannot go far wrong.

> Take the letter to your soul that you wrote earlier, open it and read it out loud slowly and deliberately, reflecting as deeply as you can on what you wrote ...
> Now reflect: What does this all mean to you "in reality", in your life now, in the "broad light of day"? ...
> What's the relevance of all this? Indeed, in a practical sense, what's the point of all this work you do on yourself? ... [write]

---— ¶ BREAK ---—

Collective responsibility

Everything we do in our lives makes a difference not only to ourselves but to everyone and everything else. Until fairly recently in human history it would have seemed unthinkable, on moral as well as practical terms, to imagine that what even the collective totality of humankind can do could make a really appreciable difference to our home planet. Yet now we realise that everything we do not only makes a difference, but those things we do carelessly and selfishly can put the lives of all the creatures on this planet in jeopardy.

We have evolved into "planetary people" and to fully honour this growth we have to take responsibility for our individual actions and the actions of our race as a whole. Everything we do can make an enormous difference, from that single squirt of an aerosol spray, a thoughtless post on social media, to closing our eyes and ears to the plight of many our fellow human beings, let alone the even sorrier plight of many of the other species of life on this planet who, in reality, have an equal right to be here.

Both our knowledge about what is happening in the world around us, with its wars, disease, disharmony and ecological imbalance, and a sense of inner inadequacy, can make us believe that there is nothing we as individuals can do to change the world in any way. When we connect with our innermost nature with a sense of self, however, we find we are also connected to everyone and everything else. We are part of a collective consciousness that is totally inclusive and infinitely caring. Realising we are a part of this collective shows us that everything we do does make a difference.

Some of the more spiritual connections we make in psychosynthesis practice can help us realise that all life forms, not just human beings, are part of a totally interconnected and inseparable energy field. While most of us may spend a large part of our lives imagining that we are separate and disconnected, once we start to explore the deeper aspects of our being we discover the underlying truth of our connection. We may not be able to "be there" all the time, indeed it may not be right for us to stay in such a state, but once we have the intimation of its real existence, once we actually experience it in ourselves, there is no looking back. We have "set our sights" on the clarity and connection that comes from such realisations, and we try to make each move we take a step in that direction.

When we realise that we are connected to everyone and everything else, we start to have a different perspective on time and space. In reality we are no less connected to an ant on a distant island in the South Pacific than we are to our noses! While it may be very rare for us humans to realise this connection, we can start moving our awareness in that direction. We can start to cultivate within ourselves a sense of this global consciousness. We can realise our individual consciousness is a small but significant piece of the total consciousness of life on our planet.

Many of the exercises and techniques of psychosynthesis can help us have an inkling of this awareness and, perhaps more importantly, ground this awareness in our everyday lives. When we ground this awareness, it helps us take actions that move the total collective consciousness forward in its positive evolutionary path. It is not an exaggeration to say that one small act made by one individual at one moment in time can make a profound difference. When we care for others, both those immediately within our field of awareness and activity, but also for all living and non-living things generally, we are grounding this consciousness. When we care for our environment, both locally and generally, we are also grounding this consciousness. Every conscious act we make that includes such caring furthers the cause of global awareness in this way.

We can find many different ways to contribute to this cause, and each way adds to the richness of our experience. Perhaps such awareness will bring about some cures for the ills that currently threaten not only our individual existence but the existence of life as we know it on our planet.

> Identify two opposing parts in yourself, or parts in a current conflict situation, and listen to the voice of each concerning what they want and need at this time ...
>
> Move to the clearest inner space available to you, look back upon these two parts and their wants, consider their needs, then ask yourself: "what would it be like if these two parts came together?" ...
>
> Act appropriately upon this ... [write]

The same process can be used to deal with conflicting "parts" on a global level as well as on this individual level. Try this exercise again, but this time choose a current world conflict. See if you can really identify with the opposing forces and hear the voice of each. See the point of view of each side. Then move to a new, third position outside of the conflict and ask the question: what would it be like if these two parts come together? You might not be able to get a complete picture or a total answer, but what you do understand in this way can help resolve the conflict, and you will now be able to send out a positive energy pattern that adds to the healing of the conflict.

¶ BREAK

Leadership towards self

To be awake, to be dreaming and to be asleep are the three types of consciousness that we explored in a previous lesson. Our aim is to be able to let go when appropriate and to become and remain lucid when appropriate. When we are deeply asleep, we have let go of our conscious intention and awareness. There are times when we are asleep and when we are awake when it is best to just let go to what happens, following the process of willing as it unfolds. There are other times when we are asleep or dreaming when it is more appropriate to awaken ourselves to love, awareness and choice and activate our energies. To connect to everyday soul is just that, to trust the flow of energy within us and to direct it when and where appropriate. To reach this "ideal", or to at least move in that direction, we need to become immanent, that is, alive in the here and now.

As you have already learned, psychosynthesis is not primarily concerned with transcendence, with going someplace else to avoid the realities of living. Quite the opposite in fact, for psychosynthesis encourages us to engage with the world, with the unfolding moment, to live in the present. We may have an eye to the future, and an awareness of how the past has affected us, but it is in "everyday soul" that we can find ourselves and live an engaged (and engaging) life.

We are all leaders in our lives, even if only in a latent form. To be able to lead is a profound challenge and a necessary part of our work. Leadership does not mean making people do what you want; it is more concerned with assisting the co-creative Self in the unfoldment of process. The main concern of leadership is the release of human potential while at the same time acknowledging the limitations imposed by the human shadow, individually and collectively. A true leader enables others to both break free from, and to include their limitations when appropriate. As it says in the *Tao Te Ching*, a leader only helps creatures find their own nature, but does not venture to lead them by the nose; a leader simply reminds people of who they have always been.

> Connect with how you see yourself as a leader or not ... what qualities do you bring (or could you bring) to leadership? ... what blocks the free expression of those qualities? ... how do you know? ... [write]
>
> Connect to a time or times when you were successful leading someone or something ... then remember a time when you were not successful in leading someone or something forward... and reflect: what was the difference ... [write]
>
> Now go deeper with your reflection ... what are the deeper things within you that affect what is on the surface for you? ... how deep can you go? ... how deep do you need to go? ...
>
> Go as deep as you can now ... imagine you are looking deep into a deep pool of water, past all the surface disturbances, the reflections of sky, perhaps of your own face, past the fish, clouds, all the other stuff in the pool, past all the other creatures that live in the pool, now seeing right into hidden depths below, beyond your sight, the depths that hold everything that sustains us ... and find a symbol or image to bring back to the surface ... [write]

When we consider leadership and the role we play, one of the major questions to arise is whether we as individuals have any importance or influence in the larger global field. Psychosynthesis asserts that if you follow your own life's process, you automatically play the role you must. Even if your role is to be the silent one who feels but cannot speak, you are essential to the world. You may play an unpopular or even a publicly unrecognised role but you are still playing a "leading" role in the sense that only when all roles are consciously represented can the world as a whole operate humanely and wisely.

Each role is a leading one because the world we live in is created by the tension and interaction between all its roles. Filling the role of the leader, the follower, the silent one, the wise one or the disturber is essential for the life of the community. Only when all the roles are filled and interact can the entire world discover its own human and self-governing capacity. From this perspective, leadership is beginning to take on a new and extended meaning. A leader is anyone at any moment who represents one of the roles in any given situation.

Being yourself is a political activity today, as it has always been, but nowadays it is openly acknowledged. Through our subpersonalities, each of us has many roles inside, and we are too complex to stay identified with one role for too long—flexibility in changing roles is important. The key to good leadership, however, is mostly to just be ourselves.

> Consider now these different levels of leadership and how you experience them in your life. How might you act more in a leadership role and bring more of the personhood style of leadership into your interactions with others? ...

--- ¶ BREAK ---

Being awake

This is an easy yet powerful exercise on inner and outer awareness.

> Spend at least one hour today self-consciously aware of each single task you're working on for this period. Treat each event with a combination of relaxation, reverence and the quiet awareness that, at least while you are attentive, this is the single most important thing in the world.
>
> When you notice yourself drifting off, be aware of it and allow your attention to gently turn back to focus ...
>
> As you stay focused on one valuable thing at a time, notice and acknowledge all the times you feel yourself being drawn to something else. Just let the thought and feeling pass by, don't grasp it. (For instance, you hear the tone of your phone ringing, but resist the urge to pick it up.) Don't dwell on distractions, just note them and let them go ...
>
> Later, after the time is up, write down two or three interruptions you think might deserve or need less attention than you've been allowing them. Assuming you want to remain centred and mindfully attentive on your life journey, reflect on what you can do about these distractions. ... [write]

World and self

A version of the closing meditation from lesson 2 follows, but this time with a different focus.

Reflect on a major world issue, either local or distant. Pick one, and consider what you know about it, feel about it, and sense about it ... (this may be the same issue you worked with in lesson 2 or something completely different).

Turn your attention inside and consider the issue you chose for your reflection. How did you choose it? ... Why did you choose it? ...

Who choose it? ... How do you feel about it now? ...

What does what you picked reflect of you, or say about you? ... In what ways do you project yourself into this problem? ...

In what ways do you negate or ignore your response to this problem? ... [write]

Imagine everything you have been reflecting upon is in a clear crystal bowl balanced on top of your head ... Spend some time with this, really feeling the weight of the bowl and all your thoughts and ideas contained therein weighing you down ...

Imagine the sun comes out above you. A strong ray of sunlight shines onto the bowl, evaporating everything in the bowl ...

Everything in the bowl is dissolved by the light of the sun and you feel it becoming lighter and lighter ... even the bowl itself is dissolved in the sunlight, and now the ray of light passes into your body and you feel it charge up your heart energy, opening you to energies of courage and compassion within your heart ...

Focus once more on chosen issue, just holding a word or basic concept or image that encapsulates this issue ...

Imagine a beam of light energy extends from you and passes to where it is needed for healing ... Be fully aware of the power of imagination as you send healing energy to your chosen issue ...

Imagine a network of healing energies extending over the whole planet, your healing energy interweaving and connecting with that of others ... Once more send out your good wishes or healing energy to your chosen situation ...

When you feel ready, come back to yourself, not drained but full of energy and engaged with the world ... Stamp your feet and do something really mundane to ground yourself back into your everyday reality ... [write]

--- ¶ BREAK ---

Inner and outer silence

During the course in this book, we have explored some of the many different types of meditation used in psychosynthesis, particularly reflective, receptive and creative meditation. Another type of meditation that is most useful and potent is silent meditation. While it may on the surface appear to be easy, silent meditation is in fact the most difficult to achieve. As you know, to sit absolutely silently, turning off the inner dialogues, is incredibly difficult, and physical, emotional and mental interruptions will interrupt the complete silence.

In order to escape our difficulties and all conflicts we experience individually and collectively, one way we humans have invented is, of course, meditation, but too often this is based on desire, on will and an urge for achievement, and therefore imply conflict and struggle. As the best meditation teachers assert, all effort to meditate is the denial of meditation. Meditation is the ending of thought, the turning off of the voices of our subpersonalities. It is only then that we can approach, hear and respond to the true inner voice of the Self within.

> Sit silently. don't do anything, let go of all tasks now and pending, don't be anything, simply be still, silent and empty...
>
> Continue this meditation for at least fifteen minutes, At the end of the time, note down all the things you remember that interrupted your concentration ... [write]
>
> Repeat the meditation daily for a week, each time at the end noting down the "breaks" to your concentration ...
>
> At the end of the week's work, reflect back over what it is that has interrupted your silence and stillness, and what these breaks tell you about yourself and the work you need to be focusing on for your continuing journey of personal and spiritual development ... [write]

--- ¶ BREAK ---

Congratulations

A final exercise and this course is completed. If you want to learn and practise more psychosynthesis, there are suggestions and pointers in the appendices. For now, though, let that go and do the following:

> Give yourself time just for yourself. Do something you really enjoy doing (what is it you most enjoy?) and give yourself over wholeheartedly to this activity ...
>
> Give yourself something meaningful to you to reward yourself for completing this course.

As an ancient Tibetan greeting says: may the blessings prevail.

AFTERWORD

The wisdom of psychosynthesis

We live in a world of polarities in our inner world no less so than in the outer, so our world experience is based on duality, and we are divided within. Psychosynthesis stresses that each part of the psyche is whole at core and has a part to play in our life.

Each of us is a fundamentally healthy organism in which there can be a temporary complaint or breakdown. Pain, crisis, failure and all our issues are opportunities for growth and essential to our life purpose. The emergence of previously suppressed or repressed spiritual material is usually accompanied by crisis, offering an opportunity for change and growth. Working thus within a transpersonal context reframes and confers meaning to our issues and engenders creativity and inspiration.

We are more than reactions to past conditioning and childhood development, and each of us has a discrete, realisable core self, or 'I', an unchangeable centre that experiences our different states of consciousness, including all thoughts, emotions and sensations, but in itself is none of these. Contact with the 'I' enables us to be self-directive, have a sense of purpose and an active impulse towards service.

We are controlled by everything with which we become identified, and, conversely, we can gain control of and have choice about everything from which we disidentify ourselves. Disidentification involves stepping back consciously from limiting identities, attitudes, outdated roles and beliefs to gain greater perspective and developing a capacity to make healthy, deliberate choices and to connect with a sense of life purpose and motivation.

As we become more centred on this core self, we develop the ability to control previously divisive elements of our behaviour, restructure the personality around this new core self, and realise the essential goodness in all life.

Becoming centred on the core self enables us to explore the heights as well as the depths of the psyche, contact a deeper Transpersonal Self that is universal to all life, and realise all experiences as part of a larger, collective expression of an inner spiritual nature.

Meditation, especially silent meditation and the evocation of serenity, but including reflective, receptive and creative forms, is essential for the stability of the psyche and maintaining a living connection with the Self.

Understanding of the Transpersonal Self comes not through transcendent experiences but directly through the personality and its interactions with the outer world. Spiritual and transpersonal energies need grounding both for the psychological health of the client and for the treasure such experiences can bring to our world.

Humans are interconnected and interdependent beings, each individual being part of a larger whole with local, social and global responsibility. Valuing life requires a self-commitment to act in co-operative and responsible ways.

The aim is not to reach a goal but to engage with the process of life in the spirit of inquiry.

Psychosynthesis always remains open to development.

APPENDIX 1

Further reading and training

Reading can help us acquire both knowledge and understanding about ourselves and other people. If we read in a positive and active way, it can facilitate our growth. This involves reading slowly, stopping at times to reflect and evaluate, copying or underlining important sections, reading with attention and interest, and being willing to stop when tired or bored. If we read in this active way it strengthens our concentration and our will, and may even help us grow spiritually.

There are many books which, although not directly about psychosynthesis, may make appropriate extra-curricular reading, and it can be both exciting and illuminating to find such as these. Indeed, once you are "living with" psychosynthesis, it is really interesting to see how the visions and values of this approach are seen underlying so much positive activity in the world even if in no way attached to or, as far as one could tell, even aware of psychosynthesis.

If you wanted to increase your library of psychosynthesis books, I recommend:

Assagioli, Roberto (1974) *The Act of Will*, Wildwood House
Assagioli, Roberto (1975) *Psychosynthesis*, Turnstone

[These books by Assagioli are a little dated in their language but they are very useful as reference manuals and are packed with gems to discover.]

Guggisberg Nocelli, Petra (2017) *The Way of Psychosynthesis*, Synthesis Insights
[A very thorough description and exploration of psychosynthesis including details of Assagioli's life and work. This is an essential book in any psychosynthesis library.]

Parfitt, Will (2019) *The Magic of Psychosynthesis*, PS Books
[If you want to take your study to another level, exploring and practising psychosynthesis in a wider and deeper spiritual context, then *The Magic of Psychosynthesis* is essential.]

Journals and articles:
Psicosintesi [journal from Italian Psychosynthesis Institute]
Psychosynthesis Quarterly [Journal of the Association for the Advancement of Psychosynthesis]
　　For an extensive and comprehensive list of psychosynthesis articles: https://kennethsorensen.dk

Videos:
Psychosynthesis intro with Will Parfitt:
https://youtu.be/7vgXbaVgUJ0

Roberto Assagioli & Psychosynthesis with Petra Guggisberg Nocelli:
https://youtu.be/Aw3_ETUF5R8

Further reading
If you want to read further on psychosynthesis, then I recommend the following books and articles in addition to those mentioned above.

Assagioli, Roberto (1942) 'Spiritual Joy', in *The Beacon*
Assagioli, Roberto (1953) *Into the Future*, World Union of Progressive Judaism, France
Assagioli, Roberto (1967) 'Psychosomatic Medicine and Bio-Synthesis', lecture given at the International Psychosomatic Week, Rome
Assagioli, Roberto (1973) Interview with Stuart Miller, in *The Intellectual Digest*

APPENDIX 1

Assagioli, Roberto (1974) Interview with Sam Keen, in *Psychology Today*
Assagioli, Roberto (2003) *The Science and Service of Blessing*, MGNA
Assagioli, Roberto (2007) *Transpersonal Development*, Inner Way
Assagioli, Roberto (n.d.) *Laser Lites*, MGNA
Assagioli, Roberto (n.d.) *Laws and Principles of the New Age*, MGNA
Eastcott, Michal (1979) *"I": The Story of the Self*, Rider
Ferrucci, Piero (1982) *What We May Be*, Turnstone
Firman, J. and Gila, A. (2002) *Psychosynthesis: A Psychology of the Spirit*, SUNY Press
Ford, Clyde (1989) *Where Healing Waters Meet*, Station Hill Press
Hardy, Jean (1987) *Psychology with A Soul*, Arkana
Nocelli, Petra Guggisberg (2021) *Know, Love, Transform Yourself*, Psychosynthesis Books
Parfitt, Will (2008) *The Something & Nothing of Death*, PS Avalon
Parfitt, Will (2012) *Walking Through Walls*, Kindle
Parfitt, Will (2015) 'Psychosynthesis', in *The Sage Encyclopedia of Theory in Counselling and Psychotherapy*, Sage
Parfitt, Will (2019) *The Magic of Psychosynthesis*, PS Books
Simpson, Evans [ed.] (2013/14) *Essays on the Theory and Practice of a Psychospiritual Psychology* [2 volumes], Institute of Psychosynthesis
Sørensen, Kenneth (2016) *The Soul of Psychosynthesis*, Kentaur Publishing
Whitmore, Diana (1986) *Psychosynthesis in Education*, Turnstone
Whitmore, Diana (2014) *Psychosynthesis Counselling in Action*, Sage

The following books, while not mentioning psychosynthesis, are excellent additions to a library of books taking a psychosynthesis approach.

Arrien, Angeles (1992) *The Fourfold Way*, HarperSanFrancisco
Buber, Martin (2008) *I and Thou*, Simon & Schuster
Chopra, Deepak (2004) *The Book of Secrets*, Rider
Grof, Stan (1985) *Beyond the Brain*, SUNY Press
Grof, Stan (1989) *Spiritual Emergency*, Warner
Hanna, Thomas (2004) *Somatics*, Da Capo
Hillman, James (1997) *The Soul's Code*, Bantam
Johanson G. and Kurtz R. (1991) *Grace Unfolding*, Bell Tower
Johnson, Don Hanlon (1994) *Body, Spirit & Democracy*, North Atlantic
Maslow, Abraham (2011) *Towards A Psychology of Being*, Martino Publishing
Needleman, Jacob (2003) *Time and the Soul*, Berrett-Koehler
Needleman, Jacob (2016) *I am Not I*, North Atlantic Books

Parfitt, Will (2010) *Kabbalah For Life*, PS Avalon
Perls, Frederick, Hefferline, Ralph F. and Goodman, Paul (1994) *Gestalt Therapy*, Souvenir
Wilson, Robert Anton (2016) *Quantum Psychology*, Hilaritas

Training in psychosynthesis

Sometimes it is said that psychosynthesis is "a psychology that includes the transpersonal or spiritual". For me it is more than that: if I had to describe it in this way, I'd rather say it is "a method of spiritual realisation that includes psychology". Many people use psychosynthesis for counselling or personal therapy and find it very effective. Others use it for enhancing their creative work and do not feel the need to include the spiritual realms, and for them this is most effective. Psychosynthesis is a unique method, however, in that it centres on the Self around which all else is said to cluster or revolve. When we centre on the Self, we are making a commitment to spiritual unfoldment as well as to psychological development.

It is very exciting to live within the vision and by the principles of psychosynthesis, and how we do this creates our own version of psychosynthesis. If we want to share it with others, we have to honour our personal vision of what it is and equally honour their "version" of it, too. We also have to remember that we are all teachers and leaders, and psychosynthesis is best understood and applied when it is a shared experience. Remember, too, that you already know the best psychosynthesis guide there is, and he or she is that same guide that knows you best, too—your own inner wisdom and understanding.

So where do you go from here? There are several tracks you could follow, including individual study and investigation, individual psychosynthesis therapy, attending seminars and courses aimed at personal and spiritual growth from a psychosynthesis perspective, or a full-time training as a psychosynthesis guide/therapist at a training centre. None of these possibilities need to be taken singly and, in fact, are probably best approached in the various combinations and at the appropriate times that suit your own personal evolution.

Roberto Assagioli stressed what he called the central decisive importance of the human factor, which inevitably unfolds through living interpersonal relations. There are many different kinds of counselling and psychotherapy, numerous different trainings and certificates and so on—so much so, it can be difficult to know what it all means, who you can trust, if the person is properly qualified and so on.

All the evidence shows that of most importance is choosing the right person for you. Of course, you want your therapist to be competent and to have done training, but more important is how you feel with them—ask yourself if you feel comfortable telling this person intimate details of your life; do you feel safe with them; do you like the way they act towards you; do you feel respected and heard? If you are at all concerned about a potential therapist's credentials, do not be afraid to ask them what training they have done; do they have regular supervision of their work; what experience do they have; and what is their code of ethics?

It is your right to interview a number of practitioners before making your choice (although you may feel fine about the first person you see, too); they may charge you for this initial interview—some do, some don't. There is a lot of information on the subject available on the Web, and your local library should be able to give you more literature on counselling and psychotherapy.

Many psychosynthesis centres and institutes have a "public program" that will include various workshops and seminars either on psychosynthesis directly or on particular aspects and applications. As well as introductory weekends, most psychosynthesis centres and institutes also run a "fundamentals" or "essentials" of psychosynthesis course, often of several days' duration, which introduces participants to the principles and practices of psychosynthesis. These introductory training courses are very popular and contain enough material for anyone to use psychosynthesis in their own work and life in an informed and practical way. Beyond this, many centres also have more long-term, in-depth training that often leads to a certificate of qualification or diploma in psychosynthesis counselling and psychotherapy.

Assagioli said that psychosynthesis functions in five main fields: personal integration and actualisation; therapeutic; educational; interpersonal; and social. So often these days psychosynthesis is seen as a counselling or psychotherapy training, and little enough emphasis is placed on its other applications. Indeed, Assagioli saying that the field of self-actualisation and integration being the heart of psychosynthesis clearly places it primarily as a self-help method for personal and spiritual development. If this course has sparked your interest in further training, maybe even professional training, do look around and check out what is local to you and apply the same questions to a centre, or their representative, that you would ask of an individual practitioner. If you want the best, you might well have to be willing to travel.

All this said, the psychosynthesis you have learned and practised in this book is very thorough and gives you an excellent ground for applying psychosynthesis, not only in general, but in all your specific areas of activity. Don't lessen or deny what you have already understood and integrated, and if you want to continue with psychosynthesis training, choose wisely.

Currently [as of early 2024] the following organisations and centres are well-established.

UK:
The Psychosynthesis Trust, London:
www.psychosynthesistrust.org.uk

The Institute of Psychosynthesis, London:
www.psychosynthesis.org

Europe:
EPA—European Psychosynthesis Association:
psychosynthesis-europe.com

EFPP—European Federation of Psychosynthesis Psychotherapy:
www.efpp.psychosynthesis.net

Italian Institute—Italy:
www.psicosintesi.it/home-international

USA:
AFPP—Association for the Advancement of Psychosynthesis:
aap-psychosynthesis.org

APPENDIX 2

A book map

This appendix lists the main sections in each lesson, which may help you find your way round the contents.

Lesson 1. The journey of life: a process of cycles within cycles	11
Starting the journey	13
Cycles within cycles	15
Who is here?	17
The ground of relationship	17
An autobiographical exercise	19
An organic process	19
The part and the whole	23
Wholeness and fragmentation	24
Before starting the next lesson	25
Lesson 2. Models of awareness: understanding our inner world	27
Defining who we are	28
Turning points	28
Crisis and opportunity	30
The egg of being	32
The next step	38

Sensing, feeling, thinking	39
Beyond pathology	41
Intuition	42
Summary of influences on our development	43
Global awareness meditation	44
Before starting the next lesson	45

Lesson 3. Subpersonalities and self-expression: exploring our many roles — 47

Review	48
Seen and not seen	48
The multiple personality	49
The difficulty with identifications	51
Wants and needs	52
The garden of beauty	54
Beyond conflict	55
Subpersonality and other	58
Love, will, change and maintenance	58
Appraisal	59
Subpersonalities and polarity	60
A deep reconnection	61
Before starting the next lesson	61

Lesson 4. Love and relationship: towards balance and harmony within — 63

Review	64
Self in others	64
Love and connection	65
Projection and perception	67
Mother activity	68
A living extension	69
From birth to adolescence	72
Childhood development	74
The expression of love	75
A true meeting	77
Choices to make	79
Before starting the next lesson	79

APPENDIX 2   211

Lesson 5. The child of wisdom: the inner child
  and family dynamics   81
    Review   82
    Back in the family   82
    Relating to the child within   83
    Growing the child within   84
    Revealing appearances   86
    Standing on the corner   87
    Renewal, change and return   88
    Sexuality and identity   91
    Developing meaning   93
    Into the heart   96
    Before starting the next lesson   97

Lesson 6. The art of self-identification: becoming the conductor
  of your life   99
    Review   100
    Past identifications   100
    Believe it or not   101
    The contents of consciousness   102
    An awareness meditation   102
    Disidentification and self-identification   103
    The self-identification exercise   106
    Soul and the stages of life   108
    Meditation   111
    The mirror exercise   114
    A wise being   115
    Object attachment   117
    Before starting the next lesson   117

Lesson 7. The power of imagination: living within the world
  we create   119
    Review   120
    Automatic drawing   120
    About imagination   122
    Manifesting and qualities   125
    The essence of symbols   127

The house of the self	129
The spirit of synthesis	130
Synthesis—an organic process	132
Are you you?	134
Before starting the next lesson	135
Perform your exercise!	135

Lesson 8. Purpose and the process of willing: personal
and spiritual empowerment 137
Review	138
The act of will	138
Making a decision	139
Not making a decision	139
How will works	140
The stages of willing (1)	143
The stages of willing (2)	144
The stages of willing (3) and (4)	147
Willing from the heart	149
Freedom	151
The helmsman	153
The source of good will	154
Before starting the next lesson	155

Lesson 9. The realms of spirit and shadow: exploring
the heights and depths of the psyche 157
Review	158
Heights and depths	158
Embodiment of energies	159
The images	160
Spiritual energies	160
Grounding energy	162
Being at peace	163
Qualities of the self	164
Motivation and intention	166
A bag of shadow	167
Layers of shadow	168
The ritual dance of spirit and shadow	171
Inner ecology	173
One flower among many	175
Before starting the last lesson	176
The course so far	176

Lesson 10. Acceptance and change: global issues
   and embodying leadership   179
     Review   180
     Set and setting   180
     Ongoing acceptance   181
     A question of ageing   183
     The ageing process   183
     Facing death meditation   184
     A soul letter   186
     We are all divine   186
     Wealth   190
     Care for the soul   190
     Collective responsibility   191
     Leadership towards self   194
     Being awake   196
     World and self   197
     Inner and outer silence   198
     Congratulations   199

Afterword   201

INDEX

acceptance, 179ff.
ageing, 183–184
analysis, 20, 127
anima/animus, 70
archetype, 58
    energies, 58–59
    of motherhood and separation, 69–72
Arrien, A., 17
Assagioli, R., 2, 12, 206
attachment, 101
    changes in, 100–101
    identification and, 101
    perceptions, 104
    object, 117
automatic drawing, 120–122
awareness, 6, 27ff., 43, 53, 56, 112, 123, 138, 193
    self awareness, 12, 158
    of personal self, 37
    global awareness meditation, 44–45
    and identity, 102–103
    focused, 196
    exercise on inner and outer, 196

baby, 16, 69, 70, 84
behaviour, 162, 170
    in self-perception, 48–49
    in ego identity, 72
beliefs, 68, 82, 95, 101
birth, 71–74, 187
    psychological, 73
    memories, 90
    development from, 109
blocks, 20, 22
Bly, R., 167
body, 28, 39–44, 71–75
    awareness, 14
    consists of, 24
    to experience the world, 39
    brain and, 42–43
    as vehicle for expression and experience, 44
    connecting to energies of birth, 71–72

216 INDEX

impact of trust and mistrust on, 74–75
nonverbal reinforcement, 93
in wheel of life, 109
in foreground, 109–110
sense of being "new born", 126
embodiment of energies, 159–163
breath, 6–7, 93, 184, 191

change, 58–59, 179ff.
character, 88, 168, 170
childhood, 74–75
choice, 22, 56, 77–78, 86, 101, 138, 139–140, 140–143, 144–145, 181, 201, 207
collective
  unconscious, 37
  consciousness, 112, 180, 192, 193
  responsibility, 189, 191–194
compassion, 13, 57
conditioning, 18, 22, 51, 152
conflicts, 22, 23, 47, 55, 68, 148, 198
consciousness, 35
  contents of, 102
  core of, 103–106
  states of, 104
  awakening planetary, 191–194
counselling, 206–207
creative meditation, 114.
  See also meditation
crisis, 30–32, 89
  mid-life crisis, 88
cycles, 13, 15–17, 110, 187. *See also* life journey

dance, 171–173
death, 184
  cycle of life, 15, 183
  fear of, 169
  accepting, 179, 181
  facing death meditation, 184–186
  as transition point, 187
desires, 18–19, 143–144, 145, 148
development, 6, 11, 41, 43–44, 70, 73, 82, 91, 109–111
  seven stages of, 15
  childhood, 74–75, 81

of inner child, 84–86
of skill, 145, 146
transpersonal, 182
spiritual, 188, 207
dialogue, 40
  and archetypal patterns, 68–69
  soulful, 190–191
differentiation, 28, 90, 110
disidentification, 201.
  See also identification
dreams/dreaming, 12, 104, 128, 194
duality, 131

egg diagram, 32ff., 89
  horizontal divisions of egg, 32
  lower unconscious/personal psychological past, 34–35
  field of awareness, 35
  middle unconscious, 35–36
  "inspirational flashes", 36
  superconscious/evolutionary future, 36–37
  "I" (or "self"), 37
  collective unconscious, 37
  personal self, 37–38
  shadow and spiritual dimensions, 168–171
ego, 51, 72, 89, 115
elder, 179, 183
environment/ecology, 142, 173–175, 189, 190, 193, 197
evolution, 21, 30–32, 143, 147, 161
existential, 89. *See also* inner child

family, 41, 66, 73, 81ff., 131
  revisiting family of origin, 82–83
  back in family, 82–83
  child, 83–84
father, 55, 82
fear, 95, 169
  of judgements, 18
  of abandonment, 88, 91
  of intimacy, 91
  of death, 169
  of losing individuality, 169
  of success, 170

feelings/emotions, 28, 39–41, 95, 101, 105, 107, 108, 127, 140, 160, 174, 184, 185
    "I" (or "self"), 37
    projection, 68
    emotionally identified, 102
field of awareness. *See* consciousness
freedom, 151–153
future, 11, 24, 33, 34
    evolutionary, 36
    child of, 87–88

global awareness, 44–45, 179ff.
good will, 149–151. *See also* will/willing process
    source of, 154–155
grounding, 23, 148, 202
    mystical experiences, 120
    energy, 162–163, 167
    desire, 166
    aim of, 167
    consciousness, 193

harmony, 132–134
healing, 197–198
heart, 18, 96, 149–151
higher unconscious, 36, 88, 164, 169

"I" (or "self")/witness, 20, 37, 43, 110, 115, 201
identification, 100–101. *See also* self identification
    past, 100–101
    and attachment, 101
    "chosen", 101
    disidentification and self-, 102, 103–106
identity, 134–135
illumination, 36
imagery, 123, 124, 129
imagination, 119ff., 135
    role of, 119
    harnessing imagination for transformation and growth, 119–120
    automatic drawing, 120–122
    transformative power of, 122–125
    "image junkies", 123
    symbolism, 123
    manifesting and qualities, 125–126
    essence of symbols, 127–128
    house of the self, 129–130
    transformative journey into basement, 129–130
    inner house, 129–130
    transpersonal Self, 130
    spirit of synthesis, 130–132
    groups, 131
    illusion of duality, 131
    creating harmony within ourselves, 132–134
    synthesis, 132–134
    essence of identity, 134–135
    expressing the "you" within, 134–135
incarnation, 28, 41, 44, 74, 90, 187
individuation, 13, 70
inner child, 81ff., 97
    nurturing, 81–82, 84–86, 93–96
    healing past wounds and embracing wholeness, 81–82
    inner subpersonalities, 82
    relationship dynamics, 82–83
    revisiting family of origin, 82–83
    reconnecting with, 83–84
    healing through reflection, 83–84
    relating to child within, 83–84
    developmental phases and healing wounds, 84–86
    growing the child within, 84–86
    self-expression, 86–87
    connecting with, 87–88
    existential and mid-life crises, 88–90
    journey of self-discovery, 88–90
    liminality, 89
    differentiation and integration, 90
    self-discovery and integration, 91–93
    sexuality and identity, 91–93
    negative patterns, 92
    developing meaning, 93–96
    path to soul integration and self-discovery, 93–96
    sense of rightness, 95

unconscious constructs, 95
assumptions, 95–96
journey of healing and wholeness, 96
reflecting on interaction with, 100
inner guide, 100, 115, 116
inspiration, 36, 188
integration, 12, 27, 47, 90, 100, 110, 115, 147, 157, 183, 207
intention, 166–167. *See also* will/willing process
interconnectedness, 191–194
interpersonal, 65–67
introjection, 64–65, 68–69
intuition, 28, 42–43

leadership
   personal, 180
   towards self, 194–196
learning strategies, 5–6
left brain, 42
life journey, 11ff.
   integrating self-discovery and holistic growth, 11–13
   "living with", 12
   reflective meditation, 13–14
   starting, 13–14
   life's cycles and patterns, 15–17
   personal development and change, 15–17
   mindful break, 17
   reconnecting with self through awareness, 17
   basic principles, 17–19
   ground of relationship, 17–19
   autobiographical exercise, 19
   psychosynthesis, 19–23
   journey into wholeness, 23–24
   part and whole, 23–24
   synthesis of self, 24–25
   wholeness and fragmentation, 24–25
   deepening your engagement with psychosynthesis, 25
love, 58–59, 63ff.
   -type subpersonality, 56
   and connection, 65–67

expression, 75–77
element, 76
lower unconscious, 34, 35, 36, 51, 105, 168, 169, 170

maintenance, 58–59
maps/models, 32ff., 84, 90, 171
meaning, 93–96
meditation, 111, 202
   reflective, 13–14, 113
   on unity and integration, 23–24
   global awareness, 44–45
   exercise, 102–103
   receptive, 113–114
   creative, 114
   facing death, 179, 184–186
   silent, 198
memory, 108, 159–160
middle unconscious, 35–36
mid-life crises, 88–90
mind, 6, 17, 35, 102, 107, 108
mindfulness, 12, 163–164
mother, 63, 68–69, 69–70, 73, 181
multiple personality, 49–50

nature, 21, 94, 189
negative patterns, 92
next step, 28, 38, 148
   guide for, 61
   inner guide and, 115

oneness and separateness, 72–73

pain, 30, 85, 101, 170, 201
parents, 65, 74, 85, 86, 101
past, 11, 12, 24, 29, 32, 34, 151, 169
   child of, 87–88
   identifications, 100–101
peak experience, 157, 159
personal/personality, 137, 190–191. *See also* subpersonality
   growth, 27–28
   self, 37–38
   multiple personality, 49–50
   "core personality", 51
   quality evolution, 57

adapted, 72
leadership, 180
personal self, 37–38. *See also* self
polarity, 60–61, 90, 181
potential, 23, 33, 43, 86, 119, 120, 133, 138, 151–152, 159, 169
power, 56, 59, 124, 125, 149, 169–170. *See also* will
process, 12
  of cycles within cycles, 15
  organic, 19–23
  of evolution, 30–31, 32
  of identification, 40
  of birth, 72
  meditative, 113
  synthesis, 132–134
  decision-making, 137
  of willing, 138ff.
  repression of the sublime, 169
  ageing, 183–184
projection, 64–65, 67–68
psychology, 11, 206
psychotherapy, 207
purpose/intent, 27, 29, 41, 74, 90, 137ff., 147, 148, 152, 187–188. *See also* will

qualities, 23, 31, 56–58, 105, 113, 119, 125–126, 154, 164–165

receptive meditation, 113–114. *See also* meditation
reflection, 82
  healing through, 83–84
  soulful, 186
reflective meditation, 13–14, 113
relationship, 63ff., 79. *See also* inner child
  subpersonalities in fictional worlds, 64
  projection and perception, 64–65, 67–68
  relationship patterns, 64–65
  principles of interpersonal psychosynthesis, 65–67
  love and connection, 65–67
  nurturing right relations, 65–67
  dialogue and archetypal patterns, 68–69
  mother activity, 68–69
  living extension, 69–72
  BPM Model, 70
  adapted personality, 72
  ego, 72
  birth to adolescence, 72–73
  oneness and separateness, 72–73
  "oral phase", 73
  childhood development, 74–75
  nurturing trust, 74–75
  expression of love, 75–77
  wholeness in relationships, 75–77
  "ideal relationship", 77
  deepening connection, 77–78
  true meeting, 77–78
  choices to make, 79
  nurturing self and relationships, 79
  dynamics, 82–83
responsibility, 191–194
right brain, 42
ritual dance, 171–173

self, 20, 28, 43, 103, 138, 157, 165
  -acceptance, 183–184
  -actualization, 138–139
  -consciousness, 103
  core, 20, 99, 201, 202
  -knowledge, 179
  leadership towards, 194–196
  personal, 37
  -development, 43–44
  -discovery, 88–90, 91–93, 93–96
  -expression, 86–87
  -integration, 47
  sense of, 64, 75, 86, 91, 162
  unattached, 89
  world and, 197–198
self identification, 99ff.
  balancing identifications and embracing core self, 99–100
  reflecting on interaction with inner child, 100
  changes in attachment, 100–101

past identifications, 100–101
reflections on identification,
    100–101
beliefs and choices, 101
"chosen" identification, 101
identification and attachment, 101
liberating the self, 101
contents of consciousness, 102
disidentification and, 102, 103–106
awareness and identity, 102–103
self-consciousness, 103
awakening to, 103–106
liberating core of consciousness,
    103–106
states of consciousness, 104
journey to self-realization, 106–108
development and integration,
    108–111
mapping soul's journey, 108–111
soul and stages of life, 108–111
wheel of life, 109
"I", 110, 115
meditation, 111–114
connecting with inner guide/wise
    being, 115–117
object attachment, 117
reflecting on attachments, 117
Self, the, 11, 20, 28, 37, 43, 49–50, 56, 57,
    106, 130, 131, 134, 147, 165,
    202
    spiritual, 37
    hidden aspects of, 60–61
    liberating, 101
    house of the, 129–130
    will of, 148
    Self and superconscious, 164–165
sensations, 14, 22, 24, 36, 37, 39, 68, 100,
    101, 111, 124, 127, 182, 201
separation, 70, 72–73, 89, 173, 174, 179,
    181
service, 112, 165, 202
sexuality, 91–93.
shadow, 51, 157ff.
silent meditation, 198, 202
skilful will, 145, 146. *See also*
    will/willing process

soul, 28
    mapping soul's journey, 108–111
    and stages of life, 108–111
    qualities, 165
    letter, 186
    soulful reflections, 186
    care for, 190–191
    soulful dialogue, 190–191
spirit, 157ff., 176–177
    "I", 157
    life's peaks and troughs, 157–158
    spontaneous spiritual experiences,
        158
    heights and depths, 158
    embodiment of energies, 159–160
    images, 160
    spiritual energies, 160–162
    spiritual emergence, 161
    anchoring to earth's core, 162–163
    grounding energy, 162–163
    being at peace, 163–164
    connecting to eternal self, 163–164
    mindful peace, 163–164
    journey to the self, 164–165
    qualities of the self, 164–165
    Self and superconscious, 164–165
    spiritual realms in psychosynthesis,
        164–165
    bridging intentions with actions,
        166–167
    grounding transpersonal energy,
        166–167
    motivation and intention, 166–167
    shadow bag, 167–168
    depth and complexity of shadow,
        167–171
    egg diagram, 168–171
    layers of shadow, 168–171
    "regular shadow", 169
    "repression of the sublime", 169
    ritual dance of spirit and shadow,
        171–173
    human ecology and
        interconnectedness, 173–175
    inner ecology, 173–175
    blossoming in stillness, 175–176

guided visualization of growth, 175–176
reflection and integration, 176
spiritual emergence, 158, 161
stages of life, 99, 108–111. *See also* life journey
strong will, 145. *See also* will/willing process
subpersonality, 47ff., 61–62
    for harmony and growth, 47
    self-integration, 47
    inner terrain, 48
    inner cast, 48–49
    and role dynamics, 48–49
    seen and not seen, 48–49
    multiple personality, 49–50
    naming and understanding, 49–50
    "core personality", 51
    "ego, the", 51
    "shadow, the", 51
    "top dog", 51
    difficulty with identifications, 51–52
    identification and integration of, 51–52
    inner ensemble, 52–54
    wants and needs of, 52–54
    garden of beauty, 54–55
    conflict and transformation within, 55–58
    love-type subpersonality, 56
    evolution of personal qualities, 57
    depths of love and relationship, 58
    archetypal energies, 58–59
    Love, Will, Change and Maintenance, 58–59
    appraisal, 59
    and polarity, 60–61
    deep reconnection, 61
    embracing diverse aspects, 61
    integrating inner self, 61
    in fictional worlds, 64
superconscious, 36–37, 164
symbols/symbolism, 123, 127–128
synthesis, 132–134
    spirit of, 130–132

thinking, 28, 39–41, 42, 55, 76, 102, 105, 109, 110, 127. *See also* mind
time sharing, 40
transcendence, 194
transpersonal
    psychosynthesis, 21
    Self, 37, 43, 49, 56, 130, 147, 202
    qualities, 56
    energies, 160–162
turning points, 28–30

unconscious
    personal psychological past, 34–35
    lower, 34–35
    middle, 35–36
    higher, 36–37, 164
    collective, 37
union/unity, 57, 59, 92, 103, 131, 132, 174

victim, 30, 100, 137, 140, 143–144, 166, 181

wealth, 190
wheel of life, 109. *See also* life cycles
wholeness, 23–25
will/willing process, 58–59, 137ff.
    stages of will, 137, 143–149
    power of will, 137–138, 140–143
    source of will, 138, 154
    steering course of self-actualization, 138–139
    act of will, 138–139, 140
    making decision, 139
    recalling essence of successful will, 139
    depths of will, 139–140
    six steps of will, 141–143
    liberation from victimhood, 143–144
    cultivating willpower, 144–147
    strengthening strong and skilful will, 144–147
    aspects of will power, 145
    exercises in will, 146
    strengthening your resolve, 146

"being will", 147
conscious realization to spiritual attainment, 147–149
evolution of will, 147–149
"true will", 148
will of the Self, 148
"good will", 149–150
activeness and passivity in will, 149–151
cultivating good will, 149–151
freedom, 151–153
helmsman, 153–154
source of good will, 154–155
wisdom, 183, 201
child of. *See* inner child
witness, 20, 37, 43, 110, 115, 201
wounds/wounding, 81, 85, 90, 181
world issues, 197–198. *See also* global awareness

Milton Keynes UK
Ingram Content Group UK Ltd.
UKHW032331231124
451543UK00013B/446